Passion

A Salon Professional's Handbook for Building a Successful Business

Susie Fields Carder

Printed in the United States of America

Published by
Carder Creative Enterprises
2713 Loker Avenue West
Carlsbad, California 92008

ISBN #0-9650777-8-0

Fourth Printing

Cover Design and Illustration:
David Lynch Graphic Design 888-282-0440

Author Photo:
CeCe Canton 619-265-2423

Contents

Foreword to 10th Anniversary Edition i

Dedication iii

Introduction vi

Section 1   Passion: Getting It, Keeping It and
Communicating It 1
What is Success? 2
The Secrets of Success 3
Super Tips from Success Makers 7
Super Confidence:
Making Your Dreams Come True 9
A Set of Values for Every Achiever 18
Is My Life Full? 19
Life and Mountain Climbing 21
Attitude: The Essential Attribute for
Success 22
Checking your A.Q. 22
Effective Communication Is
Built on Effective Listening 25
Communication and Success 27
Passionate Listening 29
How to Improve Your Listening Skills 35
In Summary 37

Section 2   Professional Presence:

Sharpening Your Image 39
That Sixty Second Decision 39
From Rags to Riches 40
Model Makers: Choosing a Role Model ... 45
Knowing the Right Words 47
Changing What Needs to Be Changed 49
Fashion Personalities: Designing A
Special Look 51
Success is Just a Handshake Away 54
How Far Will You Go? 56
Preparing a Presentation 58
Nine Keys to a Professional
Presentation 62
Don't Let It Ring Twice:
Professional Telephone Skills 63
Thank You: The Note That Counts 67
In Summary 69

Section 3   Goals: Making A Mole Hill from That

Mountain 71
Set 'Em High: Goals and Achievements ... 74
A Self-Evaluated Test for Goal Setters 76
Goals: List Method 76
Goal Summary Sheet 78
Goal Supplemental Sheet 79
Goal Summary Sheet 81
Supplemental Summary Sheet 82
Goals: Bubble Method 83
Notes On Goal Achieving 84
Focus on Business 86
Spending Plan: A Checklist to
Check Your Finances 89
Financial Checklist 90
Financial Points to Ponder 93
Getting a Handle on Money 94
In Summary 96

Section 4 Marketing: Crashing Through to Sales
Success 99
Planning Your Work and Working Your
Plan 100
Winners' Words to Remember: 104
Defining Your Plan 105
Sales Savvy 105
Top Points in Selling 110
Retail Equals Retention 111
Unique Selling Philosophy 113
Ten Commandments of Superior
Customer Service and Retention 115
Client Retention 116
Marketing Practices That You Need 117
Promoting Yourself and Your Company 121
A Sure-Fire Promotion 124
Promotional Planner 125
Leadership and Followship: Seven
Characteristics 126
The Ultimate Test of Time 127
Do It, Delegate It, or Dump It:
A Jolt in Time Management 128
Booking Strategies 133
Working Smart 135
Making Time 136
Some Salon Professionals Are... 137
In Summary 138

Section 5 Building Your Dream Team 139
Definition of Team Players 141
Building a Solid Foundation 142
From Cold to Hot: Tips on
Getting Your Team Together 147
Keeping Your Team in the Game 150
Caring for Your Contacts 152
Team Etiquette 153
A Final Team Challenge 155
An Open Letter 156

Making the Right Connections 157
Referrals: Worth Their Weight in Gold.. 159
Decide to Network 162
Praising Your Team and Your Clients ... 163
Your Praise and Recognition Challenge 167
Handling Difficult Clients 167
In Summary 169

Section 6   Passion Plus: Tips, Recommendations
and Affirmations 171
More to Think About 172
Visualizing Success 173
Affirmations 176
Promises for Well-Being 177
In Summary 178

Recommended Reading 179

Foreword to 10th Anniversary Edition

It's been ten years since I first wrote this book. I was traveling in Brazil when I came up with the title. My husband and I were on a 24 hour bus ride, feeling somewhat delirious at the time, and thinking about what the name of this book would be.

When we came up with *Passion,* I immediately knew that it described what I felt was one of the most important aspects of success. Soon after the book was published, I opened up a salon and called it Passion, as well.

Everybody I hired to work in the salon read this book and it became our Bible. Everything that I talk about in this book is what we did ourselves and four years later my salon was included in American Salon "Salon 200," as one of the fastest growing salons in the country. I was honored and it reinforced that the simple business concepts that I put together for this book, work.

Over the last ten years, hundreds of people have come up to me and told me that this book changed their life. It gave them the direction and inspiration to go out and cause their own success.

I feel so fortunate to be able to support and impact so many people in this industry. I feel blessed that I was chosen and that I chose to do something with my Passion. I have traveled the world and built a training company that delivers business trainings to nearly 10,000 salon professionals each year.

I am so proud of my team and their commitment to improve this industry. Our companies bold statement is, "Global Leaders Delivering World Class Business Education," and that's who we are. They get up early and leave late. They jump on planes nearly every weekend to teach, train, and share some of the business principles outlined in this book.

They are committed like me to giving people in the salon industry the tools to succeed and everyday I marvel at their love, their teamwork, and their friendship.

Ten years later my dream is still the same. That you enjoy the book and it helps you to create and live your dreams. If I can ever be of support, don't hesitate to email me @ susie@salontraining.com.

Dedication

Dreams do come true. The book you hold in your hands right now started as a dream and has evolved into so much more. It is my vision. It is my quest. It is the sum of all the parts that have become me. It is the reality of my passion. It is my gift for you and every salon professional in the industry.

In the beginning, I held my vision high. I had to show the universe who I was. In the process, the book has materialized. In sharing my hopes and wishes, goals and aspirations, I feel humble and proud in the same instant. I am timid and yet fearless.

All I have experienced as I present this book to you could not have been possible without the ever-supportive people with whom I am proud to encircle my life. Some have coached, some have mentored, some have teased, some have listened (and laughed) and some have hugged as we've cried. In stormy times, they've been there; in moments of peace and celebration, they've been there. I am truly blessed and thank you all.

Thank you to my right arm Linda D. for editing, supporting, correcting, and making me look like a genius. My mentors Anne Boe, Barbara Geraghty, Dr. Barbara De'Angelis, Jean Braa, Shawn Hite-Harris, Joan Lakin, Chalea Pierce, Robyn Litt, Joy Lanoue, Sharyn Tolle, Sherry Musser, Andrea Carter, Rebbecca Evans, Princess

Tina, Tasha Nelson, Bonnie Dean: Thank you for being powerful women with vision enough to share. Pat, you have been an amazing contributor to my personal and professional life. Brian Reiss, thank you for holding up a mirror and sharing in the greatness of every venture with your enthusiasm and outrageous self-expression. Moshen, thank you for standing in a place, strong with commitment, as you strive to make a difference in this industry and work toward increased prosperity for salon professionals. To all the women in Women's Impact Network and my colleagues who have encouraged me, saying, "You *can* do it," thank you. Without your support and belief, I would have still been saying, "Well, maybe someday." To Landmark Education, thank you for having a support system and educational curriculum that allowed me to see what was possible. To wordsmith Eva Shaw, a blessing in my life and my intuitive sidekick, you brought my word, ideas and dreams to life with passion: Thank you for sharing your talent and inspiration.

Dad, thank you for being a great leader. And thank you for teaching me the ethics of life and that if I wanted something I'd have to work hard. You taught me lessons that have been indispensable, including the fact that hard work pays dividends. Through example and words, I learned about paying my dues, about honesty and about integrity. I mastered the complexities of the Golden Rule, and I now know it is the basis for everything. I am honored to have been and continue to be your student.

Auntie Em, without you and your support I would have never had the courage to take many of life's risks, including attending cosmetology school. You're a risk taker and I'm gratified to have learned so many things from you; thank you for always being "mom." I love you.

Saving and savoring the best for last has always been a fancy of mine. Thus, it is with overflowing indebtedness and intense love that I dedicate this book to Bert Carder, my friend, business partner, confidant, soulmate and wonderful husband. Thank you for being so unstoppable as I continue my quest, as I live my dream. Thank you for being such an unselfish, joyful reason for my every breath. I love you. And to Amanda and Megan, my beautiful daughters who are gifts from God, I love you both. You have been my cheerleaders, my life preservers, and my reality checks. You've taught me how to be a kid, put up with my stuffy business persona, and tickled me with humor, wit and immense insight.

I love and appreciate all of you. Bless you.

Bless you, my dear friends and colleagues as you undertake a journey to capture passion. This book is dedicated to you.

Introduction

Do you remember when you first entered the industry? What did it feel like? Take a minute and think back. Do you recall the pride you sensed at accomplishing your goal — to be a full-fledged salon professional? It felt wonderful, didn't it?

For many of us, that sense of fulfillment, the dignity of our profession, has been put aside. There are always "should'ves" and "could'ves" lurking inside our heads. Have you ever thought: "I should have gone to work at one of the up-scale salons instead of this home-town shop?" Or: "I could have made more money (had more clients, given more demonstrations, been more successful) if I only had the same opportunities as Mary (or Bob or Diane).

If you've ever felt or voiced these excuses, you're in good company. Eight out of ten salon professionals say that they've been disappointed as professionals at one time or another *in the last five years*. Actually, statistics take this feeling of loss a step further; most people are unsatisfied with their chosen careers.

The great news is that *nothing is wrong*. You're okay. You're very normal. I remember working nights at a local restaurant until I built up my clientele. I thought: Why am I working so hard? What am I doing? I should just go get a real job, one job. If I had quit, I wouldn't be able to share this knowledge. How many times do we quit when success is around the corner?

You're right if you're thinking that we have all missed opportunities, possibly taken the wrong fork in the road. And we've all thought sometime in life that somebody else's grass was greener. This is common. We've all had a sense that we're only realizing or using half of our potential. What really separates those who can't shake those anxious sensations and those who acknowledge them and then move out of the career doldrums is *passion*.

Is passion missing from your professional life? Let's get personal for a minute, and give this concept some thought. I so strongly believe that we should all have passion for our business that I'll make this promise: If after you have read this book, applied the principles, and accepted the how-to's I've outlined you do not increase your success and self-esteem, I will never bother you again. No guilt. No hassle. No reminders of the should'ves and could'ves.

If you're missing passion, you're missing the boat for success and fulfillment in all facets of life. Take a second to look at this term, and see how it applies to those who work as salon professionals. In our field, passion is lust for excellence. It's a hunger for success. Passion is knowing what you do is important. Passion can be an obsession, a yearning to be your best self yet. This attitude, however, does not include comparing your career motives (or your personal goals and objectives) with others. Passion is in you and for you. You own it; yet if it's lost, you can regain it. We're all very fortunate in that respect.

Throughout this book, we'll continue to talk about passion. Using the advice contained here, you will have the opportunity to control your own destiny and recapture your passion.

Let's make something crystal clear. We each have our own road map to arrive at the point called success. But, keep in mind that we each color success with different shades of crayons. Winston Churchill said that success is moving from failure to failure without losing momentum. While you're formatting just what passion is for you, curb any tendency to compare what you want out of life with the gal or guy at the next station or next salon. That won't work.

Making comparisons only undermines self-confidence, but learning from the success stories of people with passion can inspire you. Therefore, I've included advice to motivate you on your journey toward success. I'll give you quotes to ponder and suggestions to ingest. I'll give you concrete ways to attract and maintain clients, to present yourself to your best advantage, to network, and to make more money. We're going to talk about being a professional, communicating for success, increasing retail rewards, setting goals, marketing, team building, planning for the future and visualizing your dreams. Throughout the book, I refer to you, the reader, as a salon professional. This was done to make reading easier; please understand that "salon professional" includes everyone in the salon or connected to it such as nail technicians, make up artists, colorists, perm technicians, salon owners, hair designers, receptionists, shampoo assistants, manufacturers, distributors, and salon consultants.

To make this book easier to read in quick snatches, a necessity in the busy life of any salon professional — I've organized it into short chapters. That way, you can read one in a spare moment or perhaps a section when you have a few minutes.

No one is going to make a fuss if you decide that a recommendation isn't right for you. It's okay. We all have times when we're in the "gathering stage," that is, a time to reflect and map out future plans. If you're not ready to move out and ahead, don't fret. This book will help you when you are ready. Each chapter has gotten me where I am today; a small piece of the bigger puzzle.

Nonetheless, just as I made a promise to you that you can regain your passion, you must make one for me. All I ask is that you read the advice that's shared and do so with an open mind. These techniques and methods work; men and women in the salon industry from San Diego, California to Bangor, Maine have used them to increase their:

- ✄ Communication skills
- ✄ Personal satisfaction
- ✄ Self-esteem
- ✄ Financial options
- ✄ Choices for personal and professional growth.

The stumbling blocks to achieving a higher level of success, hurdles that may have contributed to your loss of passion, probably originated somewhere in the past. The steps toward regaining your passion and moving toward success (as you define it) are available now. Your desire for success is restricted only by the intensity of your passion. Your passion is controlled only by your depth of imagination and creativity.

Here's the catch: You must promise to try to regain it or to capture it. That's all I ask. Period.

I'm a salon professional, too, and have a busy clientele as a hair designer. I've worked in salons that have great clients and wonderful teams and some salons that didn't measure up. I've been in this business since 1983, and I built my business being a single mom of two girls. I've struggled with the ups and downs just like you. I truly share your concerns and fears. But, I also believe that if you're going to do something, and take the time to do it, you should do it well. I believe that to be the best for ourselves takes commitment — takes passion — and it starts inside.

Have you ever tossed a pebble into a still pond? Passion is like that pattern of ripples. You feel successful, you take steps to become more successful and you know what? Others suddenly see you as a highly confident individual, and the ripples make a wider circle. They can alter your entire "pond" of life *forever*.

Motivational speaker Brian Tracy asks, "If you could dare to do anything in the world, and there were no limitations, what would you dare to do? What would you dare to be?" Are you ready to take on that dare — to be the best, to be passionate and to be the most confident person you can be? No need to wait — turn the page, and let's get going.

Section 1
Passion:
Getting It, Keeping It and
Communicating It

Do you have what it takes to really succeed in our highly competitive field? It takes passion. By examining passion more closely, it's easy to see that it's full of possibilities and even more secrets. In order to unravel the meaning of passion, we'll focus on the secrets of success and professional presence immediately, since it is the foundation on which to build a successful career and a more fulfilling life.

In this section, we'll disclose the secrets of becoming even more confident, ways to measure your personal satisfaction and thoughts that might just change your attitude.

Since presence is more than who you want to be, we're going to look even deeper at the personal secrets of a successful life. Presence is a blend of your inner-most self and the self that the world meets, so we'll also focus on your professional image with tips and suggestions on the power of communicating, listening, and shaking hands.

Additionally, I believe there are clients everywhere. So we'll focus on skills to attract new clients whether we are at a network meeting, club meeting, church meeting or professional mixer. Therefore, I've included information on how to plan a presentation.

I think the best "secret" in this section, however, is the power of saying thank you. How often do we forget to credit, recognize, and acknowledge those who are important to us, the individual at the next station, the person who delivers our products, our clients, and our families? Proclaim yourself a rarity in this hectic society, and learn great ways to say "You're important. Thank you so much." There's no time to waste. The secrets of success and passion are waiting to be revealed. Do we have any time to lose? Definitely not!

What is Success?

To be successful, realize that:

There is no such thing as standing still.

Time lost is time gone forever.

Life lessons are valueless unless we've gained insight.

The Secrets of Success

Here, ready for your immediate use, are some of the best secrets of success ever formulated. It's a formula you'll want to use every single day of your life. Remember, just as easy as they are to do, they are easy not to do, too.

1. *Keep smiling.* It's hard not to smile back when a smile comes in your direction. With a smile, you can change a person's mood or improve a person's day.

   Secret Note: Your face can't tell the difference between an honest, spontaneous smile and one that is put there to make others happy. Smiling feels good; it makes others feel good, too.

   Try this right now. As you read the next few paragraphs, put your lips into "smile position." Don't you feel better? Of course. Make smiling a habit to transform your world for the better.

2. *Avoid arguing.* Never disagree with a client. You're not going to win. End of story. While the client may not be correct, that aspect hardly matters. You are not winning a war, and you're not the captain of the high school debating team. This person is your client; this person is your business.

   Secret Note: When a problem arises, look the disgruntled customer in the eyes, acknowledge what has been said, and reply, "What I understand you to say, Tina, is that you are angry because..." or, that "You're upset because..." or, "How can I make this better for you?" Listen to the response, and use positive body language, such as, a smile, erect posture, a firm handshake. If possible, end your question with Success Secret #1.

3. *Give a minimum of three compliments each day.* Every person wants recognition; some of us need it more than others. Have you ever said something like: "Hey, Bert, great shirt," and watched Bert beam. Or, "Kiki, that last weaving you did was spectacular." And Kiki's reaction? Smiles, and quite possibly, the receiver stands a little taller.

We all need compliments, and I've found that when we give them, we get them back. Make a personal effort to give three sincere compliments each day.

If you stay with behavior-based compliments such as "You're always on time," or "I appreciate your knowledge and artistry," people generally have an easier time believing you. The behavior-based compliments make you seem more sincere versus trial-based compliments, such as: "Your eyes are pretty (or your blouse is stunning...)."

Secret Note: There are endless possibilities to meet your compliment quota. In addition to those people in your salon, you can give compliments in your personal realm, too. Did the grocery bag person carefully place the bread at the top of the brown sack? Did your significant other or offspring do something helpful without even thinking that he or she was doing you a favor? Was a sales clerk, bus driver, school teacher, postal worker, garage mechanic or other service person especially friendly, courteous or kind? Does that give you a few ideas? Yes, these folks and other people in your life will give you perfect opportunities to reach your quota.

4. *Make an effort to reach out and touch someone.* The customer relations office with the New York City

Public Libraries recently did a study concerning non-intrusive touching. The librarians found that when they made contact with patrons in non-intrusive ways — a pat on the hand, a finger's touch to the elbow, and so on — patrons reported that they had received more caring and helpful service than from non-touchers. The patrons believed that there was a connection to the public servant, and they felt a warm bond to the library that they couldn't quite explain. Nonetheless, they gave the library's customer service survey higher marks.

Take some advice from a librarian, and create your own bond with clients. Although we're in the high-touch business, we need to extend that technique to immediately greet clients.

Secret Note: With your next three customers: 1) Shake hands. 2) Pat a shoulder. 3) Touch an elbow. 4) Or you can do as I do, and hug each client. I always feel better when I share hugs, and my clients admit that they do, too.

5. *Mirror positive emotions and behavior.* Does your client seem to bubble with happiness? Mirror that. Is your client excited? Get your excitement level up. Is your client subdued or introspective? Put the bubbles and excitement aside, and make it a time for quiet conversation.

    Secret Note: You can move mountains with this one secret alone. Be sensitive and empathetic. Make your emotions genuine.

6. *Use your client's name often.* While you're providing services or selling products, use the client's name frequently. "Barbara, how was the traffic getting here?" "You know, Brian, you must have been on vacation;

5

you look so tan (or relaxed or fit)." We love our names, and feel good when others use them. I believe that there is nothing more beautiful than the sound of our own names, and using names is an easy "success secret" to include in your every day business.

Secret Note: Make your goal to use a client's name a minimum of seven times during the appointment.

7. *Make eye contact.* Look into your client's eyes when listening. Let them know what they're saying is interesting, and you're very interested. If you're not, you'll probably lose that individual as a client.

Secret Note: When using a client's name in conversation, make sure you're also making eye contact.

8. *Cultivate your sense of humor.* Read funny books. Go to funny movies. Tell at least two jokes a day. Remember, good humor never offends — make sure your humor is inoffensive.

Super Tips from Success Makers

While gathering information for this book, I talked with the movers and shakers — the really passionate people of our industry. I asked questions like a nosy two-year-old-child, and I got a bundle of advice on what one needs to be successful. Here's the best of the bunch. Circle your favorites. Adopt at least three pieces of advice today:

- ✄ Keep moving.
- ✄ Keep trying.
- ✄ Give the gift of heart.
- ✄ Get off to a good start in anything you do.
- ✄ Give your enthusiasm to everyone.
- ✄ Be yourself.
- ✄ Forget yourself.
- ✄ Become genuinely interested in the other person.
- ✄ Be fair, honest, and friendly, and you'll be admired and liked.
- ✄ Make others feel important.
- ✄ Count your assets, and stamp out self-pity.
- ✄ Put your smile power to work.
- ✄ Meet people on their own level.
- ✄ Keep your temper to yourself.
- ✄ Work smarter, not harder.
- ✄ Keep your promises.
- ✄ Learn from the examples of others.
- ✄ Overwhelm people with your charm, *not* your power.

- ✂ Forgive yourself if you fail.
- ✂ Be lavish with kindness.
- ✂ Be a do-er, not a say-er.
- ✂ Count your blessings.
- ✂ Don't keep score — nobody really wins.
- ✂ Laugh at yourself.
- ✂ Share.
- ✂ Think twice before you give unwanted advice — or any advice.
- ✂ Look for the good in all people and every situation.
- ✂ Be an optimist.

"I don't know anyone who has got to the top without tenacity. That is the recipe. It will not always get you to the top, but it should get you pretty near."

— Margaret Thatcher,
former Prime Minister of England

Super Confidence: Making Your Dreams Come True

Never say "fail"

Have you ever said or even thought, "Gosh, I'm a failure." I believe that your mind can only go one direction at a time — either in the positive "can do" way or the opposite direction toward failure.

This "F" word, failure, could actually be sabotaging your success. Those who have confidence will not even think about using this "F" word and rightly so.

About five years ago, University of Southern California professors Warren Bennis, Ph.D. and Burt Nanus found out in their study of 90 highly successful leaders, the super-confident people "simply didn't think about failure — they didn't even use the word."

The study showed that the confident people acknowledge errors, but they used synonyms such as glitch, bungle, setback. They viewed their blunders as miscalculations. They did not fail, but rather used these as learning experiences to help them avoid future fumbles.

Patty, the super-confident owner of an up-scale San Francisco salon, recently made a wrong decision. She honestly revealed the significance to me in order to share this story with you. The price tag? It cost the salon nearly $100,000. Ouch!

I asked, "Patty, how do you feel about the loss? Do you feel awful about losing so much money?"

Patty simply shrugged, and replied, "Perhaps I should have, but I don't. To me, money is just a way of keeping score in the game of life — and I'm sure I'll regain my score. More so, I've always believed a mistake is just

9

another way of doing things. We learn a whole lot more from what doesn't work than what does." Summarizing her philosophy, Patty quotes actress Sophia Loren: "Mistakes are part of the dues one pays for a full life."

Trust your ability to learn

When offered a chance to do a job we've never attempted before, many of us protest: "I don't know if I can do that. Maybe you should ask someone else. I've never had experience in that area."

In case you haven't realized it before: We're not born knowing everything. But we're born to learn as much as possible. Smart people — the super confident men and women of the world — continue to learn and to seek out learning as part of their daily lives.

People who have mastered the super-confidence game wade right in. They figure what they don't know, they can learn. Early in her career, Gloria, a prominent stylist in the Dallas/Fort Worth area, won a contest offered by a manufacturer. The prize was to assist the luminary Vidal Sassoon with a demonstration at a national beauty show in New York. Looking back, Gloria remembers, "If I'd been holding a handkerchief, I would have been twisting it wildly trying to make up my mind. I'd never done anything like that before. I was born and grew up in this tiny, dusty town in southwest Texas. Why, I'd never even been east of Houston."

Today, Gloria chuckles with a contagious laugh, "Somehow I managed to say thank you and that I'd love to assist." It was the best thing she could have done for her budding career. She explains. "Weeks before I was to go to New York, I learned everything I could about being an assistant — all the etiquette. I talked with the producers of the show about what would be expected of me. I badgered the product line distributor with questions, and I learned. I even arranged to stay with some friends of friends who promised to help me navigate Manhattan. Then, I read everything I could on body language and presentation skills. Sure my time on stage would only be a few minutes, and I knew I was going to be there to assist, not provide the instruction, but I take work seriously."

As luck sometimes has it, Gloria never did assist Mr. Sassoon. Rather, something better happened. Because one of the platform artists was suddenly called away, Gloria was asked to fill in. "Had I said, 'No' to the initial invitation to go to New York, I would never have made that super confident leap. I probably wouldn't have gotten the courage to move to Dallas — or strut into the foremost salon in the city to ask for employment. If I hadn't made that leap, I may never have realized my dream of working with dignitaries, celebrities and other exciting people."

Honor yourself

As children, we're taught that it's not nice to brag, talk about ourselves constantly, and crow about our accomplishments. Boasting still isn't good form, but honoring our accomplishments is a different ball game. From this moment on, do yourself a favor and honor your successes. Love yourself, and feel proud.

Lucille Ball, that incredible actress, once said, "Love yourself first, and everything else falls into line. You really have to love yourself to get anything done in this world."

If we love ourselves, we're proud of our accomplishments. This doesn't mean that we should flaunt a humon-

11

gous tip or tell the world why we got such a hefty raise. It means personally congratulating ourselves on a job well done and enjoying the moment by savoring it.

Publicly, you might say, "Thank you so much — I couldn't have done it without everyone's help." Privately, crow all you like. Jump up and down. Scream a little if you like. Hug yourself, and say out loud that you're a winner. And as you slip off to sleep, you might want to recount exactly how glorious it felt when you pulled off that incredible success.

Every night before I slip into bed, I write in my success journal. I write down everything I am proud of myself for, and what I did that was terrific. I have even shared this with my daughters and asked them to name one happy thought or thing that went well that day. You'd be surprised how hard this is. It seems easier to focus on what we didn't do.

Downplay your mistakes

People who have super confidence accept that they make mistakes, however, they don't dwell on them, over-dramatize them, or personalize them.

Running out of gas on the way to work doesn't make you stupid; it simply means that you need to pay more attention to details. I once dumped a bottle of color down a client's face. I was humiliated, but I resolved it with quick action. I gave her the service free because of my clumsiness, apologized profusely and learned some amazing lessons.

Dropping a bottle of shampoo or hair color and making a mega-mess on the salon's new carpet doesn't mean you're a klutz; it means that you were probably rushed. You may need time management skills.

Lecturing yourself with "I've always done stupid things" may be based in school-days experiences. Children can be exceptionally cruel to one another, and sometimes adults can be purposefully hurtful to children. I call these the "negative or old tapes," and when we commit an "oops" in life, they rewind through our minds. They sometimes seem to be on a continuous tape so we hear them over and over when confidence is low.

According to success experts, the only way to stop the berating is to deny those thoughts and clarify ourselves as adults. We must push the off button to the stupid tapes and get rid of them. Our minds can only go to one thought at a time; choose the one you would prefer.

Sure you may have done something you wish you hadn't. Everyone does something unforeseen once in a while. Remember, this is just one incident in your entire life. It says nothing about your self worth. It says nothing about you as a professional or as a woman or man. Your best advice? Get over it, and concentrate on why you are a valuable person. Concentrate on one really great personal quality. Do you have a wonderful smile? Are you a genius with a weave? Is your checking account always in balance? Do you have a joyful home life? Great chef or gardener? Have lovely eyebrows or a way with poetry? Turn off the old tapes, and play your best quality tapes instead.

Give yourself a pep talk

Anytime we start a self-improvement program, we're nudged or perhaps obsessed as to what might have been. Here is where the "should'ves" and "could'ves" can get even the most positive folks feeling a bit down.

"If only I could've avoided eating all those goodies during the holidays, I could fit in the clothes I love to wear to the salon." "I should've listened to others (parents, spouse, kids, friends) and not invested in the salon because now money is so tight."

Personal or professional, these thoughts are an extension of the "old tapes" mentioned above. Why berate yourself? Make your self talk, your personal pep talk, positive.

When I trained with Dr. Barbara De Angelis, a relationship expert, she shared a three-step routine called the "Power Process." To use it, you look into a mirror and shout as loud as you can all the things you hate or which anger you. For example: "Susie, I hate it when you don't believe in yourself."

The next step is to acknowledge what you want. Okay, so you're unhappy. What do you need to do now? For example,

"Susie, what I want you to do is go into that business meeting and show them who's boss."

The last step is praise. Praise yourself for all the love and good you have to offer. "Susie, I am so proud of you for standing your ground, etc."

Repeat the process until the anger and frustration dissipate. You'll be surprised how hard it is to compliment yourself and acknowledge all the good. But, with practice you'll be super confident. This is probably one of the most powerful techniques I've ever learned. Best yet, you can do it anywhere you have a mirror and feel cleansed and energized.

Here are more ideas:

✂ Write what's good or positive about yourself or the situation in a success journal.

✂ Speak these affirmations in the present tense: "I am creating new relationships in my life. I am creating wealth in my world. I am able to ask for a raise (better location in the salon, more assistance, and so on).

✂ Make a cassette tape of your favorite statements — starting with "I am" and listening to it in the car, before bed, anytime you need a personal pep talk.

✂ If life seems to be getting the best of you, check the resources for some counseling or self-help groups. Reach out when you need assistance; people are there with helping hands.

You're worth it

The old adage of "you get what you pay for" is unequivocally true in our business. If you want something you must go after it and know your worth. For example, let's say that in your town the average rate for a woman's haircut and blow dry is $18. However, you do an exceptional job, and your clientele refers new customers on a regular basis. Perhaps, it's time to give yourself a raise. If you're unsure of the going rate for anything, ask colleagues, and call others salons for prices. Know your worth, and you will never underrate yourself.

Super confident people know what they are worth. They do not apologize for the fact that they are in business; they do not give their services away unless they do so with eyes wide open. This is your business, and if you want good things to happen to you, you have to ask. Remember you have to spend money to make money. When I started my speaking career, I spent more money than I made on press kits and videos and promotional supplies. I made a lot of costly mistakes, but I learned and achieved great things.

Super confident men and women get ready for success. As Oprah Winfrey once said, "Luck is a matter of preparation meeting opportunity." The folks who achieve super results make plans, continue their education, network with colleagues, and ask for business. Super confident people reach out for success, and it comes to them because they know they're worth it.

Let go of fear

"Yes, I acknowledge fear, but I do not let it rule my life," explains Chris, a colorist in Los Angeles. As a teenager, Chris immigrated to the United States to live with a distant relative in one of the tougher sections of the city. Chris worked in all sorts of odd jobs in order to save enough to enroll in cosmetology school.

"A lesson I learned early on was to feel the fear and move through it. I move on from fear — if it looks like a brick wall, I build a ladder. When I'm in a fearful period, I ask myself the 'what if's,' that is, what if this terrible thing or that terrible thing occurs. What's the worst that can happen? Looking at fear in this way, I know the odds and the obstacles." This winter, Chris will join a firm that produces a national product line and will begin teaching color at shows throughout the country.

Use the "what if's" if fear is stopping you. Experience the fear of a situation, but don't be disabled by it. Super confident people look at their options, and then break the fear down into manageable chunks. For example, if you're nervous around people you don't know, take a class at the community college on presentation skills. If you're not sure how best to dress for a specific body style or image, hire (or barter with) an image consultant to get more information. If you're designing the interior of your salon and just can't get it right, talk with an interior decorator or a student who is studying decorating. If you're concerned about saving for the future and for retirement, ask colleagues to recommend a financial planner or get some books on investing. Take charge of your fears and they'll make you stronger.

When I started building my clientele, I decided to do seminars for corporations on professional presence. I'd never spoken to an audience, but I thought: How hard can this be?

I managed to get a meeting with the human resource director at a local corporation, and she booked me the following week. The day of the presentation, I woke up from a restless night sick to my stomach. I called the human resource director and told her there was no way I could come. Bursting into tears, I told her my uncle had died.

To this day, I have no idea what possessed me to lie, but I know fear was a great motivator. Needless to say, I rescheduled for the following week. This time I was determined to go through with the plan. Again, I woke up sick, but pushed through the fear.

Fifty participants attended the seminar. I was so scared and nervous that I was surprised that they stayed to hear what I had to say. But, they did. That experience birthed my speaking career. The feeling of accomplishment left me feeling euphoric. If I had quit and let the fear take over, I wouldn't be able to do what I'm doing now.

Specialists who coach super-confident business people stress that throughout any self-improvement program, we must be kind, generous, loving and thoughtful *to ourselves*. Take baby steps before the giant steps. Give yourself plenty of pats on the back. With these suggestions and stories, you, too, can make your dreams come true.

Fear leads you to believe that where you are is a safe place and going forward is a risk. But, in fact, the truth is that you are always at risk: Risk of stagnating...risk of missing out on your destiny.

A Set of Values for Every Achiever

The greatest handicap: Fear.

The best day: Today.

The greatest mistake: Giving up.

The greatest stumbling block: Ego.

The easiest to do: Find fault.

The top comfort: Work well done.

The greatest need: Common sense.

The best gift: Forgiveness.

The Greatest knowledge: God.

Is My Life Full?

At the end of a working career, the wise person looks backs, and thinks, "I've enjoyed every day of this journey." The unhappy individual scowls, "I've worked myself to death, and now I'm too old to enjoy the fruits of my labors."

What was missing from that second person's life? Simply put, it was the joy of work. There is true satisfaction from performing a job well, and that's the joy of working. This doesn't mean that working isn't hard — that's why it's called work! Discovering joy in work, however, enables us to more fully enjoy life. It's savoring the journey as well as the destination.

Wisdom is gained by being open to all facets of life — our working life and playing time, and all the other joys that make our world unique. Sometimes we gain the most wisdom from the most difficult lessons; sometimes the most joy is experienced in the simplest situations.

Check yourself with this questionnaire. Answer: "Yes," "No," or "Sometimes."

1. Do you spend enough quality time with your children and/or family in a giving, loving and sharing atmosphere?

2. Are you involved with your community, your neighbors, your friends?

3. Do you allow for some private time every day to regenerate or regroup?

4. Are you taking care of your physical health through proper nutrition and exercise, and when appropriate, seeking professional advice?

5. Do you take pleasure in the work from which you are earning a living?

6. Are you constantly developing new skills or knowledge related to your profession?

7. Do you have a sound and workable budget for spending as well as saving?

8. Do you feel a spiritual connection and support this by regularly attending a service or through prayer or meditation?

9. Do you daily appreciate the blessings of nature with the changing of the seasons, the animals and plants, the sun at noon and the stars at midnight?

10. Do you feel at ease in your life and position?

Examine your responses. Consider that work, play and prayer all join to create a full, gratifying life.

Is your life full? By asking this question, you have made a move to change any area that doesn't seem as satisfactory as you would like. This quiz looks simple, but the answers can produce extraordinary changes in life if you give them a chance.

Life and Mountain Climbing

Here's a thought to ponder:

Live your life each day as you would climb a mountain. Occasionally glance toward the summit. This keeps your goals in mind. Look down toward your feet as you climb higher and higher, and partake of the beauty so close at hand.

Marvel that each step on your journey produces a new vantage point. Climb slowly and steadily. Savor each passing moment. Know that the top is in sight.

And the view from the summit? It becomes an uplifting climax for your journey, but it isn't the entire journey. Every step you took brought you to that point, and without each step you wouldn't have made it.

Your life and your world are what you make them by your thoughts and your deeds.

— Author Unknown

Attitude: The Essential Attribute for Success

Discounting luck and rich relatives, what's the character-istic that makes one individual succeed and another flounder? It's *attitude*. The really great news is that a positive attitude can be acquired.

Attitude is how we face our job, how we face our responsibilities, and how we accomplish everyday activities. It is the motivating force behind our wanting to continue to do and to be the best we can be. It is our desire to handle every situation with a professional manner in a positive way. It's picking up the pieces after a shattering experience and gluing our lives back together. Attitude is facing every situation with optimistic anticipation.

Do you have a positive mental attitude? People who cultivate passion in their lives certainly do.

Checking your A.Q.

Passionate people say that attitude is everything in life. The individual who knows all the professional skills and tech-niques, but doesn't have the motivation to use them is no better than the person who doesn't know any of the how's and why's. Knowledge is only useful when it is put into action with the right attitude. The attitude of a professional toward a career must be one of commitment to serve, whether the salon or client or both.

What is your Attitude Quotient — your A.Q.? Let's check it, and find out. The following list may help analyze your attitude. The more times you can honestly answer *always*, the better your attitude is for achieving success in the salon and out.

Passion: Getting It, Keeping It and Communicating It

1. I am enthusiastic.

2. I am self-motivated.

3. People often comment that I have a optimistic and hopeful outlook on life.

4. I follow through on all my promises so people know they can depend on me.

5. I am confident and not easily discouraged.

6. I use my cassette player to listen to educational, sales and motivational tapes.

7. I accept constructive criticism graciously because I want to improve.

8. Creative problem solving is one of my strong points.

9. I am willing to try fresh methods.

10. I have the persistence to follow perplexing undertakings to completion.

11. I work well with others.

12. I am aware and sensitive to the needs and wants of other people.

13. I strive to act like a professional at all times.

14. I steer clear of idle gossip and negative chatterboxes.

15. I communicate well with my superiors, peers, and subordinates as well as with family and friends.

16. I am well organized.

17. I believe planning is an important aspect of success.

18. I can think quickly in difficult circumstances.

19. I am proud of my ability to use common sense.

20. I seek additional educational opportunities in and out of the salon or company.

21. I really believe in what I am doing and that I am important.

22. I keep a manual or file of useful ideas and suggestions, success strategies and tactics. I refer to it, and add to it often.

23. I read at least one motivational or inspirational book each month.

24. I enjoy finding new applications for my personal computer and/or ways to streamline my work in order to better serve my current and prospective clients.

25. I incorporate laughter into every day, and use it to dissolve tense situations, if appropriate.

26. I seek ways to praise people.

27. I know that if I love what I do, and do the best I can, the money will come.

28. I plan for my future through a regular saving or investment program.

29. I am open to time management techniques.

30. I consider myself a valuable person.

What's your A.Q.? Could you answer "always" as much as you wanted to? If you're hesitating even a little, review the list. Turn it around, and make this attitude quotient into an affirmation list. It will give you 30 passionate ways to improve your attitude.

> *"Living the past is a dull and lonely business; looking back strains the neck muscles, causes you to bump into people not going your way."*
> — Edna Ferber

Effective Communication Is
Built on Effective Listening

To communicate means to be understood. For salon professionals, it is a skill that is potent. Being a good communicator can have a positive influence on life; conversely, being an ineffective communicator can keep one stopped in his or her tracks.

While there are many factors woven together to form the patchwork of your path to success, communication is an integral component. Effective communication is the act of purposely responding after listening. Listening is more than hearing; it's putting a meaning to the sounds we experience. Listening is the ability to receive, connect, attend to, and interpret verbal and non-verbal clues to what is being said or demonstrated through body language.

Are you aware that we have different communication and listening styles? Experts who design customer satisfaction programs for corporations have broken them down into these different ones: discernment, comprehension, evaluation, empathy, and appreciation. Every listening experience includes all five. Here's how the five styles work:

Discernment: The purpose of the discernment phase is to gather complete information. The discerning listener focuses on the main message and decides which details are important.

Comprehension: The purpose of the comprehension phase is to organize and make sense of the material and information. The comprehending listener relates what is being said to his or her personal experiences and attempts to understand the relationship between the ideas.

Evaluation: The purpose of the evaluation phase is to focus on making decisions based on what has been said. Evaluating listeners ask questions, contemplate motives, and accept or reject the messages according to his or her personal beliefs.

Empathy: The purpose of the empathy phase is to support the speaker during the conversation or presentation. The empathetic listener accepts the message as it is being presented, without prejudging it.

Appreciation: The purpose of the appreciation phase is to relax and enjoy what has been said. The appreciative listener gets into the moment and can easily be entertained, informed and inspired.

Allow your natural talent for listening, and your desire to be a great communicator, develop. Have a willingness to hone your skills to actively and positively reach clients, team members, and others on your journey to success. Try to overcome communication barriers by being aware of how you are listening.

By understanding each type of listening style, you can close the communication gap. I like to play a game when I meet someone and try to evaluate which type of listener he or she is by actions and words. It keeps the conversation interesting and helps me to sharpen my skills.

What can be achieved through better communication and better listening? Client trust and retention. It's as simple and complex as that.

Communication and Success

Do you realize only 15 percent of our financial success is technical ability? That leaves 85 percent of our work place success dependent upon communication skills. However, some of us are better communicators than others.

Experts in communication say that of the mistakes made in business at least 75 percent can be attributed to lack of clear communication. The next time you communicate with a client, really listen to what he or she is saying.

If you don't understand or if you want to make absolutely sure you understand what is being communicated, repeat the statement made or ask questions. You will be considered a professional and a caring person. Try this technique even when you believe you're communicating clearly. The results may be surprising.

Anyway

People are unreasonable, illogical and self-centered,
Love them anyway

If you do good, people will accuse you of selfish, ulterior motives,
Do good anyway

If you are successful, you win false friends and true enemies,
Succeed anyway

Honesty and frankness make you vulnerable,
Be honest and frank anyway

What you spent years building may be destroyed overnight,
Build anyway

People will really need help but may attack you if you help them,
Help people anyway

Give the world the best you have and you'll get kicked in the teeth,
Give the world the best you've got anyway.

— From a sign on the wall of Mother Teresa's Shishu Bhavan, the children's home in Calcutta, India

Passionate Listening

What's the easiest way to distinguish a successful salon professional from one who isn't? Simply watch how they interact with their clients.

See the one who is doing all the talking, never letting the client get a word in edgewise? Nine times out of ten, you'll be looking at the individual who can't seem to make it in our highly competitive profession.

In order to put passionate listening to work, you must allow clients (and all the potential clients in your extended network) to speak. You must let others talk about themselves and to curb your tendency to monopolize the conversation. Why? Because you'll receive valuable information.

Allowing your opinions to steamroll through a conversation or merely overpower another person rather than show how you can help is a sure-fire way for you to lose a client and lose business. If you use a hard-sell technique with your clients for products or services, you jeopardize your future. Additionally, if you're only "people pleasing" and never really provide the professional advice clients want, you'll lose out, too.

When I started my business in 1983, I was excited and anxious to share my life with my clients. After all, I had a captive audience. Looking back, I can't believe I still have some of those same clients. Now I do most of the listening, and I ask a lot of questions. I ask clients about their needs, wants and desires. My clients feel I am appreciative, and I really care.

Keep in mind what the writer Anne Morrow Lindbergh said, "The most exhausting thing in life is being insincere."

Use your professionalism, and you'll sincerely please your clients and yourself.

To be sure, you and I believe in our profession and the products we use and sell. Most of us think that what we do helps clients develop better self esteem and a more confident appearance. Regardless of how strongly we believe in ourselves and our service, we have to listen, not lecture.

Listening is the only way to target the service or product with the unique set of concerns the client presents to us. By remaining focused on helping the client — rather than making a sale — we build trust. Trust is crucial in building a successful business.

Passionate listening doesn't just mean paying attention to the client's words. Only a portion of what we actually communicate is verbal; actually 55 percent is non-verbal. It's the nod of a head, the smile, wide eyes, etc. It is essential to listen in such a way that you maximize every opportunity to pick up non-verbal cues. By doing so — giving the client the time to make an important point — you'll stand out from the vast majority of service people who simply talk too much.

Passionate listening means that you'll provide services and sell products that you believe are in your clients' best interests. You must establish yourself as an expert, and then live into it — that's why clients come to you for advice.

For instance, Beth, a long-time client, called for an emergency appointment to have her luscious auburn curls cut short. These were the same curls she had nurtured and conditioned for the last few years so I was surprised by the call.

Sitting in my chair late in the afternoon, Beth said, "Susie, I just have to have a different look — short and efficient — especially now that I have this great new job. It's the executive position I've been training for. Curls just don't belong in the board room," she concluded with a sigh. The sigh was an important clue in our conversation as was that slight frown she made at the end of the sentence.

I listened to her words, but I also knew my client was coming for advice. Yes, I could have cut her hair short and made it look exactly like the photo in the magazine she brought. But I believed that she needed to examine other options — that's what a salon professional does when he or she really listens.

"Okay, Beth, I understand that you need a competent, businesslike hairstyle, but don't you love your hair around your shoulders when you're not wearing a suit and silk blouse? Let me show you some styles that are easy to create and give a strong career look."

You've probably guessed the end of this story. I didn't cut Beth's hair that day, even though that's what she initially wanted. Today, it's longer, and more beautiful than ever. Rather, we spent the next hour braiding, twisting, sculpting, and designing styles that fit her new position in corporate America, without cutting one curl. Best yet, Beth knows how to recreate all the styles at home in the brief time before scooting the kids off to school and herself to the office.

Getting down to basics, a salon professional doesn't sell his or her service, but rather we help. We're problem solvers, and we have the answers. That's why we continue to take classes and stay abreast of the newest fashion information. Our goal is to pass along important information. After clearly demonstrating how the product or service can help achieve an objective for the client (more manageable hair, an easier-to-handle style, etc.), the final decision is made by the client — not us. Ideally it's best to know what it will take for the client to accept the product or service offered, and then let the client sell him or herself. This is what happens by passionate listening.

P.J., a thirty-year veteran stylist in the Milwaukee area, owns a bustling salon that caters to the twenty-ish generation. It's such a successful shop that the retail products constantly have to be restocked. Here's how P.J. and others explained the right way to listen:

- ✂ When your client or potential client wonders something aloud, give him or her enough time to complete the thought.

- ✂ Don't jump in right then, and interrupt. He or she may need more time to think.

- ✂ When asked pointed questions, do your best to answer succinctly.

- ✂ Listen for the reaction in both verbal and non-verbal ways.

- ✂ Allow the speaker to complete sentences.

- ✂ Never interrupt, but let the speaker interrupt you any time he or she wants. Stop your thinking process to make sure you're listening.

- ✂ Express genuine interest in the things the speaker is saying.

- ✂ Keep one ear and both eyes tuned to the subtle messages the speaker is projecting.

All this sounds easy, but most of the techniques that passionate listeners use must be practiced. Here are other points to ponder as you strive to improve listening skills.

✂ When you talk or give a demonstration or presentation, don't go on and on. Keep an eye on your client to make sure what you're saying is interesting. Change the octave of your voice, and keep a smile on your lips. If what you're saying isn't interesting (and you can always tell if they're really listening), change gears. Ask questions about the problems the client faces because you're probably missing something. Never become hostile or combative with the client.

✂ The first ten or fifteen seconds with a new client will determine the quality and length of your relationship. This is because there is an intangible, feeling-oriented "sizing-up" phenomenon that occurs early in any new relationship — including the distinctive, intimate one between client and salon professional.

✂ Much of who you are and how you are perceived as a communicator — brash or retiring, open or constricted, helpful or manipulative — will be on display in a subtle but crucial manner in those first moments. Make sure you are sending the messages you want to send.

How are listening skills improved? Here's an outstanding idea from Tracy, a salon owner in the Miami area. She explains that she always takes notes during the first few minutes of consultation time with a new client. Why? "It dramatizes the situation, and tells the client I'm so intent on pleasing him or her that I'm taking notes to refer to later. It also shouts the fact that I respect the client's needs." If you think it is impossible to listen and take notes at the same time you're wrong — the two actually reinforce each other. Just jot the concepts down using key words; don't try to record every sentence the client says.

Once the conversation has begun to pick up some steam, go back to your notes and discuss what you understand the client to have said. Ask the client to expand on key concerns; ask for clarification if needed.

Okay, I can hear you. You're saying: "Well, that's fine in theory, but what if the conversation is going nowhere? How do I listen if there's nothing to listen to? Shouldn't I take over the conversation?"

Probably not. The odds are that early in the first meeting with the new client you simply do not know each other well enough to discuss what the client really wants. Instead, focus your questions on three simple areas: The past, the present, and the future. For instance you could ask, "What specifically did you like about a favorite hair cut (color, perm, etc.)?" You might say, "What are your present needs for a style (color, perm, etc.)?" And you can ask, "What are your future plans for your hair? Do you have any long-term goals we should work toward?"

It will be up to you to add the "how" and "why" where appropriate. That's all you usually need. Take notes on the responses.

After you've listened passionately and talked with the client, you'll be ready to discuss in more detail what you can do to solve the client's problems. Remember, God gave us two ears and one mouth for a very good reason. Use those ears passionately as you create a listening environment for success.

How to Improve Your Listening Skills

So many people are so impressed by the sound of their own voices and opinions they miss wonderful opportunities to learn, acquire new attitudes, and enjoy friendships, as well as gain important business connections. In social conversations, you may miss something crucial if you talk too much; in a business setting, you may lose a sale. The salon professional who actively listens to a client's needs and actively seeks ways to satisfy the client winds up at the top.

Here are some time-honored and successful how-to's on listening:

1. Limit your own talking. You can't talk and listen at the same time.

2. Be interested, and show it. You must convey a genuine concern and a lively curiosity. This encourages clients to speak freely so you can better understand their needs, desires, and viewpoints.

3. Tune in to the other person. Are you giving your full attention or is your mind wandering? Concentrate by practicing to shut out unwanted distractions.

4. Think like a client. Clients have important needs. When you better understand the client's viewpoint, you will retain that client.

5. Ask questions. If you don't understand something or feel that you've missed a point, clear up the confusion. Your lack of understanding could embarrass you later.

6. Hold your fire. Plan your responses only after you are certain you have a complete picture of the client's viewpoint. Prejudging is dangerous. A pause, even a long pause, doesn't always mean they've finished speaking.

7. Look and listen for buying signals. Remember to focus on key, hot-button comments. In our dealings with others, we must be knowledgeable of prime motivating factors. Once we have identified these factors, we can gently push their buttons to get the response desired.

8. Listen for ideas, not just the words. You want to get the whole picture, not just isolated bits and pieces, so make sure you're listening to the ideas and concepts.

9. Use interjections. An occasional "yes," "I see," or "Is that so..." shows the clients you're still there, but don't overdo this technique or use the words as meaningless comments. A client can tell when you're really paying attention.

10. Turn off your own worries. This isn't always easy, but personal fears, worries, and problems unconnected to the client form a kind of "static" that can blank out the client's message.

11. Prepare in advance. Remarks and questions prepared in advance free your mind for more active listening. Prepare a list of what you want to discuss or the suggestions you want to make.

12. React to ideas, not to the person. Don't allow irritating things people sometimes say to let you become annoyed. We all have rotten days, and you don't know what's really going on in your client's life. You want to strive to be a peaceful person with a calming influence on others.

In Summary

Throughout this section, we've focused on sparking or rekindling the passion for our profession. Here are some key points to remember:

- ✂ Passion is communication
- ✂ Passion is investing in our future
- ✂ Passion is having strong ethics
- ✂ Passion is having the right attitude to succeed
- ✂ Passion is listening, active listening

In the next section, we'll investigate ways to sharpen your image, to face the world, and to understand how the world perceives you. If you're in the market to dynamically improve your career, continue reading.

Section 2
Professional Presence:
Sharpening Your Image

That Sixty Second Decision

Do you realize that when you meet someone (or see someone again after a long absence), an opinion is formed about you in the first 60 seconds? Only 60 seconds and a judgment has been made.

The person you're meeting assesses your educational background, economic status, and intelligence level. More so, he or she may even make a judgment call on the type of car you drive, the highest grade of post secondary education you achieved, and if you're married, single or available and looking. This person also makes a decision as to whether he or she should do business with you. All that is determined on just the way you look and talk in the first minute of your relationship.

Let's talk about this 60-second decision making process. What decisions are your clients making about you in that brief initial encounter? Are you professionally dressed? Are you able to communicate your ideas in an articulate way? Do you show empathy? Are you dynamic without being abrasive? Let's discover each of these parts of the professional presentation puzzle, and see how your pieces fit.

From Rags to Riches

The importance of a successful image for the salon professional is typically underestimated or overlooked. Remember those 60-second decision making processes when a new client walks into your salon. What does he or she see? Are you clean and neat, but in t-shirt and jeans? Are you cutting hair or doing nails in a dress or a shirt and slacks that have seen better seasons? If you answer "Well, just once in a while," you're undermining your success. You can justify it, but remember, it's a game called success. The one who knows the rules and the plays like a professional wins. That's really the bottom line, isn't it?

Want to make more money? Then begin to create your own power to pick and choose your clientele. How does one do that? You can do a lot toward making more money by simply sharpening your professional image with what you wear to the salon.

I did not always like dressing up to go into the salon. I never liked wearing pantyhose. I didn't wear business attire unless I had a business appointment. But perhaps like you, I wasn't entirely satisfied with all my clients. I wanted to offer more upscale services; I wanted to cultivate clients who were comfortable spending from $30 to $150 without batting an eye lash. While chatting with my mentor about this topic, the light suddenly turned on in my head. If I wanted a better clientele, I had to look and act more successful. Thus my quest began.

After making the decision to give myself and my ideas a make over, I took my professional image seriously. I planned the steps it would take, and I put the plan into action.

I put away the jeans (even the ones with the "right" label on the back pocket); I shoved those comfortable and roomy casual clothes to the part of my closet reserved for leisure-time outfits. I really took the plunge and decided that I had very little that was appropriate to wear for this new business venture.

Without spending a fortune, I carefully selected the basic pieces of my new professional wardrobe. Just like you can do, I built it around a few classic, high-quality items. Then I blended the pieces with items from my closet. For example, I wore a short and snappy black wool skirt (new) with a creamy silk blouse (from my closet) and added a designer scarf (new) with geometric designs to make up a great professional look. I wore the small gold earrings that I'd had for years and a plain gold watch. I was striving for understated elegance. That outfit worked and became one in which I felt very comfortable.

(I also began to and still do wear a black apron over my clothes to protect them from the chemicals and sprays that are part of our world. Yes, I do manage to ruin a few things, but the investment in business clothes and the right aprons is well worth it.)

As I began acquiring clients who wanted more expensive services, I invested more money in my business wardrobe. The transformation took over six months to complete because I initially had to carefully budget my clothing allowance. Did it work? Absolutely — it was like giving myself a raise, and it increased my income by 50 percent in just one year.

As I found out recently, studies indicate that women who wear makeup, have their hair professionally done, and wear a business-style clothing earn an average of ten percent more than women who do not. With slight changes in the description, that goes for men, too. Actually, I believe that figure is far too low. I think that salon professionals can dramatically see an increase in their income with this suggestion alone — dressing for success counts. This difference is a statement we make, and a loud statement it is, that we are professionals and desire to be treated as such.

Now it's your turn — let's look at you. If you're over 17, you already know that fashion styles come and go. What's "in" is a state of mind, and it goes out about as fast as we change our thoughts on the subject. Therefore, when investing in your professional wardrobe, select classic styles, and brand names that will ensure you'll be able to wear the garment for more than one season. I like great flashy looks, but I also demand that the clothing be well made and comfortable for a full day's wear in the salon.

I know what we do and what we wear in our private life is our own business, but when marketing to the professional environment, it's essential to look like a professional. You need to think about how a professional sees you and perceives you. Now if you're targeting people in the twenty-ish age group, your "dress code" may be more casual, but clean and well kept, nevertheless. It's tough to go wrong with business attire regardless of the clientele.

Now a few words in favor of stockings. If you are a woman who chooses to wear a dress or suit, you have no choice — you must wear stockings. To do otherwise is tacky. Sure, I hate them just as much as the next woman, but stockings promote a professional look. Shop around for stockings, and make your choices from pantyhose that slim, tighten and trim to hosiery that stops thigh or knee high. If you need to wear stockings that provide support, find the most sheer ones possible. Always wear hosiery that fits, and make sure it's in good condition. Unsightly snagged or sagging stockings, like clothing that's too tight, could ruin your professional image.

Generally, selecting a color that matches your shoes will give a slimming appeal. One stylist I know always wears taupe shoes, and yes, always wears taupe panty hose. It's a "together" look that fits her well.

Now let's look at *your* hair. When was the last time you had your hairstyle changed? Or your hair color enhanced? How do your nails really look? Are they manicured at all times? Or do you have chipped nail polish or rough cuticles, or no polish at all? These sound like small things, but your clients notice. Take my word for it.

Skin care experts always say: Put your best face forward. Skin is that important. What does your skin look like? Is it broken out? We sell beauty, and the health of your skin says a lot about the products and services you provide. Do you need to visit a dermatologist or invest in a deep facial? With technology at our fingertips, everyone can do something to create beautiful skin. The only thing that's keeping you from attaining beautiful skin, quite possibly, is lack of information. You owe it to yourself to make your image as sharp as possible.

Cosmetics can make a world of difference in how we face the public. The top models who sport the natural look spend about two hours to achieve that appearance. If your make up skills are rusty or outdated, seek some professional advice within your salon or out. Talk with a make up specialist, and determine your goals as you design a make up program you can live with.

How about your shoes? How do they look? Do they need some repair or polish? Are the heels scuffed or blackened from the rubber mat near the gas peddle of your car? Impeccable shoes reflect your image of perfection.

Like you, I'm on my feet all day so I choose a brand of leather pumps that the manufacturer swears could double in comfort for sneakers. On the topic of high heels, some salon professionals do, and some don't. If they're your cup of coffee, then heels are fine. I agree that they look great with suits, but if you're like a lot of us, low-heeled shoes fit your needs better. The choices in low-heeled pumps are extensive and still announce that you're a business person. While you're investing in your professional wardrobe, you may need to purchase two new pairs of shoes in neutral colors so you can wear them everyday.

The key for your professional image is to dress in a way that you model the outfits your clients wear or the prospective clients wear. Remember, likes attract likes.

Now that you're getting the package well put together, let's look at accessories. Jingles, bangles, and fun jewelry is just that, and in moderation, it is alluring. However, you must choose accessories with care if you want to attract a professional clientele. Jewelry should produce compliments and comments, not distract clients.

Last, but hardly least, let's talk about your body. If you're over the weight at which you feel most comfortable, it's time to do something about it. Starvation, unbalanced, or crash diets don't work — they never have. The only real way to reduce unwanted body fat is through regular exercise and a low-fat diet. Support groups and weight control programs can guide you. There is help as close as your phone book if you're over your comfortable weight.

Achieving a fit body is more important than the numbers on your bathroom scale. When we're fit, we have more endurance and are better able to handle the stress of those 12-hour days that salons are so famous for. I highly recommend beginning or continuing on a sensible fitness program. Your stamina, flexibility, and energy level will increase, and you'll be perceived as a passionate go-getter. You'll probably seem five years younger, too, because energetic people seem youthful.

Model Makers: Choosing a Role Model

Who do you admire? If there is someone in or out of our profession that you admire, ask yourself why. If appropriate, perhaps it's time to emulate that person. Even without personal advice, your role model can act as your mentor, and you can rationalize how he or she will dress, speak or act in any situation.

For example, Phil, a hair-cutting genius in the Washington, D.C. area, greatly admires the style of actor George Hamilton. "He's suave and sophisticated. I know my clients would love to have their hair done by Mr. Hamilton — if the actor was a stylist, of course."

Admittedly, Phil doesn't exactly have George's outward appearance — Phil stands just over five foot and is built like a football linebacker. But the discrepancy in appearance hasn't stopped this entrepreneur from taking charge of his life and attracting more upscale clients.

"About two years ago, I made the decision to imitate George Hamilton's style and charm. I'd constantly ask myself: 'How would George act, talk, or present himself.' I like the way he really seems to care about people. I like his charisma, and how he can laugh at himself. And I admire how he dresses."

Apparently clients responded well to the change. Referrals increased threefold. Actually no one really ever says, "Hey, Phil, you look just like a movie star," but they do know the Phil Brothers, who not only cuts hair like a pro but has a classy personality, is a winner. Just to let you know, Phil's appointment book is always full.

If your role model is more accessible than George Hamilton, and if it's appropriate, ask for an appointment to talk with the individual. Explain your personal goals, and tell the person that you admire his or her style and business savvy. Have your questions ready, and ask for advice.

Be prepared to hear your mentor's advice. You might not enjoy all the analysis. For instance, if you ask about your professional appearance, and you're wearing shorts and a tank top, be ready to hear that the outfit isn't right for a determined business person.

You may also find your role model in the public eye. While writing this section, I talked with a number of successful salon professionals who said that they did not have just one role model, but various models as their professional presence evolved. Anna, a stylist in Seattle, explains, "When I started to turn my professional image around, I modeled my presence after the top stylists in our salon. Then I switched to one of the leading stars of styling in the industry. Recently, I've modeled my professional presence after a blend of Hilary Clinton and Demi Moore. I want to be considered a successful woman with plenty of brains and great looks, too."

I dare you to take charge of your image. I challenge you to find a mentor, model the success of the mentor, and don't let another day go by without making a change toward a more professional image.

Knowing the Right Words

Being successful generally takes more than good looks, experience and talent. Being successful requires excellent communication skills. From now on, think about every word you speak. Even with a good vocabulary, the way you communicate with clients and your professional network may say something entirely different about you.

Katrina, from the Boston area, heard me speak about professional presence, and after a seminar, we stayed in touch. Knowing that I was working on this book, we next met at a national show and talked over lunch about professional image.

Kat confessed, "I'd always felt uncomfortable about being with really smart people. My family was quite poor, and I left school at 16 to enter beauty college. I knew my word usage was narrow, and my Boston accent over-whelming. I felt embarrassed — mortified to open my mouth in public. I was weighted down by my inadequacy with well-constructed English grammar. However, I was determined to bring in a more upscale clientele and eventually open a really grand salon. I was afraid but even more distressed about not improving myself."

Kat started what she called a "renovation program." She began studying words, including those in the monthly column of *Reader's Digest* magazine. She posted her words of the month inside a cabinet at her station and used them regularly. She says, "I took your advice, Susie, and began each day by reading the front page, the sports page, and the editorials of the newspaper. I always read the comics, too, because I love to laugh. I took what you suggested, and I call it my 'success habit.'

"Reading these sections gives me plenty of contemporary, pertinent topics to discuss with clients. I immediately found out that clients would much rather discuss current events than hear gossip about so-and-so in the salon. I also copied a list of best-selling books from the *New York Times*, began at the top, and read my way to the bottom." Kat also took a giant step to gain more confidence and success and joined Toastmasters, a group that helps one another acquire public speaking skills. Groups are normally listed in the telephone book, and that's where Kat found a local club. "At Toastmasters everybody supported my need to soften the rough edges of my accent and help me change the way I pronounced words. Giving speeches — something that scared me to death — gave me incredible confidence that I now bring to my business and other facets of my life."

Language shouldn't hold you back. Kat used her precious spare time to boost her knowledge of words and current events. As she read more, she felt more comfortable quoting from the newspaper or best-selling books and using the words she'd learned from reading. By doing so, she felt more successful, took marketing chances, became a joiner, and drew more successful clients into her chair.

I think of a fluent, strong vocabulary as a form of currency. It's great to have in your "wallet," and although you don't need to flash it around, you can use it when you desire. I believe that I literally read my way to a more prosperous career. And, you can, too.

Changing What Needs to Be Changed

If there's anything in your personality, background, or education that is hindering your progress and limiting your passion to succeed, do something about it. This advice holds true regardless of the concern. Whether your worries are emotional, physical or spiritual, seek professional advice and help yourself to a better future. Like a coach who works with professional athletes, we sometimes need a life coach (a professional we contact to help with the change). This individual may have insights or experiences we have yet to realize.

I was devastated after my divorce. The last thing I wanted to do was to build my business. But the reality was: Hey, you need to make even more money to supplement your income to raise your daughters. So I sought out a support system and an amazing life coach, Larry Laveman. He helped me stay on course, clear out the past, and move forward to my future.

I learned that change is tough and requires courage. Often our family and friends are confused when we begin to live in a different way; sometimes we have to seek support from others who are more successful. If you have negative people in your life, don't buy into their negativity as you become more passionate about your upward-moving career. Most likely, they'll change for the better or fade away.

I remember looking at all the people I had in my life. How many really cared about me and my success? I took an inventory about what a friend was, what I needed from a friend, and what I could contribute to a friendship. I did weed out a lot of people, but those who are close to me now are people I can truly depend on.

After reading what other stylists have done to improve their professional presence, isn't it time to take a personal inventory of your strengths and weaknesses? Keep in mind that a minus is just an unfinished plus mark. Don't wait until "someday," because someday probably won't come — begin to turn your minus into a plus right now. Today is the day to start your change.

If you want to make a million bucks, you must talk, act, and think like someone who makes a million bucks. And you know what, if you do that, you'll feel like a million bucks, too.

Fashion Personalities: Designing A Special Look

Women and men in our profession: Don't skip this chapter — it's a must read for those of us who are befuddled about fashion. Even though we have talked about professional presence, the next step in self improvement is considering your fashion personality and the personalities of the clients you want to attract.

Here's a crash course in Fashion 101:

There are four different fashion personalities. They include the dramatic, classic, natural and romantic. Where do you fit? Are you sending out mixed signals? Let's find out.

The Dramatic Fashion Person is Dramatic Donna or Don. Both Donna and Don share a body type that is tall, slender, angular, and often the typical model type we see in fashion magazines. You probably know someone like Donna or Don from school or in your business network. This fashion type strides into rooms with gliding motions. Gestures are purposeful. The Donnas and Dons of the world tend to have slow, decisive movements. Their choice of colors and clothing includes those that are very intense and/or very high contrast — high fashion is essential. Their choice of hair styles run the gamut from severe to soft, but always in fashion. Facial features are sharply defined and normally angular. Donna and Don's are reserved, dignified, sophisticated, self-assured, and very formal. Female prototypes are women like Tina Turner, Barbara Streisand, Cher, and Liza Minelli. Male prototypes include Sean Connery, Montel Williams, Magic Johnson, Jack Nicholson, and Bruce Lee.

Classic Karen and Ken are of average height with well-proportioned figures. This fashion personality's carriage and gestures are calm, controlled, poised, and refined. The coloring for the Classic Karen and Kens of the world is light to medium and always soft. Hairstyle is controlled, softly moving, stylish but never to the extreme. Facial features are well-shaped and regular. The clothing style that Karen or Ken chooses is soft, tailored, fashionable, but never trendy or faddish. Personality type includes a tendency to be calm, nurturing, well-mannered, organized and gracious. Prototypes of the female Classic Karen are Grace Kelly, Diana Ross, Kathleen Turner, and Martha Stewart. Male prototypes include Bill Cosby, Kevin Costner, Prince Charles, and General Colin Powell.

Natural Nora and Ned have strong, well-coordinated, sturdy builds. This is the ultimate natural individual. Women may wear make up and dress in expensive fashions, but they're a natural woman beneath. Nora and Ned's carriage and gestures are relaxed, spontaneous and happy. They walk with a free-swinging stride. Coloring is light to medium and often prefers pastels. Hairstyle is natural, easy to care for, and Nora likes to blow dry the shoulder-length locks. No frills for this person. They are usually lightly tanned, often freckled and have great natural coloring. Clothing tends to be casual and includes plenty of sportswear, even though they maintain a hint of elegance. Nora or Ned's elegance is often quite obvious in the choice of evening wear — tailored but dynamite. Personality traits are warmly informal. They're known to be frank, funny and friendly. Prototypes for Nora include Oprah Winfrey, Cheryl Tiegs, Shirley MacLaine, and Ann Murray. Male prototypes include Tim Allen, Mel Gibson, Tony Gwynn, and Bill Clinton.

Romantic Rhonda is one curvy gal and her opposite in Romantic Ron is a to-die-for-hunk. Rhonda and Ron have bodies that are well endowed, soft and round. They both sometimes fight a weight problem. She's often called "voluptuous." He's called "beefy." Carriage and gestures are graceful and relaxed. Coloring is soft or intense. There's no half way point. Hairstyling preferences include curly, soft, and ultra feminine for Rhonda and with a got-to-get-my-fingers-in-it lushness for Ron. She'd never consider a classic, straight to pulled-back style; he'd never shave his head. Facial features are soft, rounded, with large eyes and luscious lashes. Clothing preferences include the flowing, European styles. Personality traits are charming and very flirtatious. Good prototypes include Elizabeth Taylor, Whoopie Goldberg, Gloria Esteban, and Ann-Margret. And when you think of Romantic Ron you have to include Elvis, Marcus Allen, Arnold Schwartzeneggar, and James Dean.

Here's your challenge. Type cast yourself and/or your client list. This is an eye-opening exercise. When we mix fashion personalities for ourselves or our clients, we can't get that "together" image. This disjointed look discredits us in the eyes of our clients and to ourselves.

When we attempt to give Classic Karen a cut or color best suited for Dramatic Donna we do a disservice to a client. We probably don't satisfy the client's desires either. We may actually lose the client if we're not aware that hairstyles reflect fashion personalities.

Get yourself together, and then look no further than your clientele to make sure you're helping them achieve the best fashion personality possible.

"It isn't until you come to a spiritual understanding of who you are, not necessarily a religious feeling, but deep down with the spirit within, that you can begin to take control."
— Oprah Winfrey

Success is Just a Handshake Away

What's the value of a handshake? It could be worth plenty to you and your business.

A handshake is one of our most important and powerful business tools. It identifies you and your level of confidence and success. It also helps to make a non-intrusive physical connection that establishes a bond with clients. Then why is it that stylists rarely shake a client's hand? That has always puzzled me. So...when was the last time you shook a client's hand?

When we shake hands, clients immediately feel acknowledged and special. On the receiving end, you show that you believe in yourself, your talents and the products you sell. A handshake is a sign of respect. It says that you respect a client for his or her knowledge and time.

Think about the last time someone shook your hand. What impression did this person make on you? A lot depends on that handshake. Isn't it time you considered how you're shaking hands? Here's all you need to know to use a handshake as one of your best business tools. Here are three examples of handshakes.

The Wet Fish: We've all felt this one. Suddenly we're touching something that is limp and flimsy, perhaps even a little clammy. Yuck! That's why I refer to it as the "wet fish" handshake. This type of handshake shouts a lack of self-esteem and a low confidence level. The handshake lasts a mere three seconds and makes you feel like you'd like to wipe off your fingers when you're finished. If you're a "wet fisher," your client may be having trouble believing in your abilities, especially if you're attempting to sell more services or products.

The Aggressor: The person who uses the "aggressor" chooses to squeeze with a vice-like grip, and he or she puts enough force into that handshake to make you think that your arm will be yanked from the socket. This handshake lasts about three minutes and utilizes a fast pumping motion. It is also extremely aggressive and intimidating, according to experts on body language. If you're using the aggressor, you probably began doing so because you wanted to seem eager, but you must draw the line before you scare your clients with your strength.

The Classic: This is the proper handshake for professionals, and it will impress people and win you new respect in and out of the salon. Make sure that when you grip a client's hand, your grasp is firm, but not tight. Let the other individual know you're there, but don't cut off circulation.

When shaking the hand, be slow and purposeful. No need to rush. Be sure to have good eye contact, acknowledge the client by his or her name and smile. You might say, as you grasp and begin a classic handshake: "Judge Smith, it's a pleasure to meet you. I appreciate your taking time out of your busy day to be here with me." Then allow your hand to fall comfortably to your side, continuing to smile. Your client will know that you are sincere, you are making him or her welcome, and you are a true professional.

Here is your challenge for the day: With your very next client, use the classic handshake. If you've used the other two, you may have to really concentrate, but it's definitely worth the trouble. Yes, success may be just a handshake away.

"The strongest principle of growth lies in human choice."

— George Eliot, from
Daniel Deronda (1874)

How Far Will *You* Go?

Where would we be if we dropped out of school the day kindergarten finished? How about elementary school? Sounds silly, doesn't it?

Then why is it that after high school or college, and our time at a cosmetology school or with an apprenticeship, we stopped our educational process? Knowledge is power, and even more so, knowledge is essential as a tool to become more professional.

Benjamin Franklin said, "If we take the coins from our pockets and invest them in our minds, our minds will fill our pockets to overflowing." Yet, if we don't invest in our minds, whether it's money or time, we will stagnate and become stale. I don't know about you, but I refuse to consider that alternative.

We can't have too much education. Education gives us the ability to unfold new possibilities and to attract new people into our lives (and new clients) because we'll speak their language. I'm not suggesting you study Spanish, Swedish, or Swahili. I'm talking about being able to intelligently discuss a host of subjects.

Consider also that our jobs are technical. We sell good feelings and solutions, but we do it in a complex world of products and services. So, the more education we acquire in our technical job as salon professionals the better we problem solve.

One way to do this is to keep yourself current on trends and advancements in the profession; be sure to use the proper terminology, too. When you speak with confidence and with eloquence about the product or service, you will build loyalty and trust from clients. If you're wishy-washy as to why someone should buy a product or service, guess what? You will not make the sale and might even lose your client.

For a minute, picture yourself in the doctor's office. You've just been diagnosed with a grave medical problem. The doctor looks up from a clipboard, and says, "Well, I learned about your condition back in medical school, and, well, I think I remember how to treat the illness..."

What would your opinion be of this doctor? Would you trust the person or value the advice? Of course not. In the same way, a client will not value your advice if you lack information and confidence.

We're like super sponges when it comes to education. Our brains have the capacity to soak up and retain new knowledge. We're really amazing creatures, don't you think? Take time to soak up information about our industry, learn and retain that information, and then be ready to share it with your clients. Many manufacturers host an abundance of educational events. It's always surprising to me that I see the same 100 people at all the events; these people are also the top 10 percent of the industry.

I invite you to look inside yourself and ask: What do I need to learn? Would you like to be a better salon professional, parent, friend, or business leader? A passionate professional contemplates personal weaknesses and focuses on turning those weaknesses into strengths. He or she breaks the big goals into smaller, workable goals and then begins. I challenge you to begin.

I believe: What you think about, you talk about; what you talk about, you bring about. What are you thinking about right now?

> *"If you deliberately plan to be less than you are capable of being, then I warn you that you'll be unhappy for the rest of your lives."*
> — Abraham Maslow

Preparing a Presentation

"Give a presentation? You're kidding. Absolutely not." That's what most people would say when asked to provide a program.

If it hasn't happened yet, there will be times in your professional life when you'll be asked to present information to a group of colleagues or clients or at a networking meeting. The choice is to flounder, flutter, and possibly faint, or proceed with the passionate confidence of a professional. Yes, I know that most of us would rather cross raging rivers in a rubber boat then stand in front of an audience, but with a few tips, your presentation will go smoothly. Why, you might even find you really like the thrill of being at the center of attention, I know I do.

In the beginning and the end...

Every good story needs a strong beginning and a great ending. When planning a presentation, keep these concepts in mind. Devise a powerful way to start; create a provocative opening sentence that sums up all you plan to cover. This is your theme, and you can refer back to it throughout your presentation.

Once you have a beginning, decide on a good way to conclude your presentation. Traditionally, speakers review the points covered, and sometimes end by taking questions from the audience. With a good beginning and a solid ending, you're more than half way to filling in the middle part of a great presentation.

In any speech, it's best to select a few main points, three or four at the most. Expand on the points with clear examples and anecdotes. You might want to quote well-known people, perhaps an industry spokesperson or a famous leader. You might want to quote some statistics, too.

If you state three successive facts, your audience will be dozing in a matter of minutes. Once you make a single point, give an example or reword the statement, illustrate it with a story, then state it again. This concept alone will provide the basis for an outstanding presentation.

What about written notes? They're okay if you really need them. Rather, you might want to write the main ideas on 3 X 5 cards which you can place in front of you and to glance at when you need them. Be aware that you're *speaking* and not *reading*. Speak to your audience from the information in your head, not from the notes on your cards.

Many successful speakers write out their entire presentation, including just where they'll put their hands, and just where they'll tell a joke at any particular moment. They rehearse the speech a number of times; some even video tape themselves to make sure they're using positive body language.

I speak on topics about which I have knowledge. I organize my thoughts, and then practice in front of the mirror. Remember, you already know more about the beauty industry than the average person because you live it. Volunteer at civic meetings such as the Rotary Club, Kiwanas, etc. These groups are always looking for speakers with new and interesting topics.

Another avenue to consider is associating yourself with a distributor. They are always looking for educators who want to give back to the industry. Most likely they will pay you a fee every time you provide a class.

After writing the speech, some speakers make another draft of the presentation and highlight the main areas, breaking the speech down into small parts. Finally, after rehearsing that portion a number of times, they write a simple outline using only key words, and keep the key words on a note card. Behold! The speech is ready, and the speaker is ready, too.

When you're presenting...

Once you have prepared the speech, relax. Feeling nervous is common. Most speakers feel this way, and some actually love that emotion because they know it gives them an extra shot of adrenaline to increase their energy level. The feeling adds excitement to the delivery. I call the emotion "stage delight," rather than stage fright.

Before you go on the stage, perhaps an hour before you'll be speaking and definitely before the group arrives, walk around the room where you'll give the presentation. Stand at the lectern or place where you'll give the speech. Close your eyes, and visualize the audience out there listening to you. Look at the chairs, the walls, the scenery outside. Straighten your posture, find a comfortable pose for your feet, and pretend that you've just given a knock-out speech. This visualization technique gives you a giant measure of confidence when you actually give the presentation. I do affirmations such as: I am a powerful speaker ... I have the information that the audience needs ... I am a fun and engaging speaker. The affirmations create the space I want to be in, and I deliver more powerfully.

After the introduction, stand, and walk to the center stage or podium. Make sure your feet are again in a comfortable position; or make sure you can walk around and still be heard. Smile, and take a few calming breaths. Always thank the audience and the person who introduced you. Then take a moment to pause and allow the audience to settle down before you begin.

While speaking, make eye contact with each person in the room. This contact should last only two seconds, and you need to really look at people. If you have a tendency to talk fast, consciously slow your words. I always make sure there's a glass of water available for me. I've never been tongue tied, but should it happen, a sip of water will allow you time to collect your thoughts.

As you reach the point of concluding your presentation, end with a short illustration, an affirmation or another pertinent bit of wisdom. You could say, "I'd like to conclude today with this thought..." Then do so. Don't belabor your point.

If there's applause, smile, and accept the praise. As Mark Twain once said, "I can live for two months on a good compliment," and, I agree. Praise feels that good. More so, consider that you've now just done something 90 percent of the people in your audience wouldn't have the nerve to do: Give a presentation. Best yet, the next one will be more fun.

"No person is more unhappy than one who is never in adversity; the greatest affliction of life is never to be afflicted."
— Anonymous

Nine Keys to a Professional Presentation

1. Speak with confidence.

2. Speak earnestly.

3. Speak with conviction.

4. Rehearse your speech in front of a mirror or friends.

5. Use comfortable gestures.

6. Use visuals such as flip charts.

7. Have fun. Laugh. It's your party.

8. Make sure you hand out your business card and brochures.

9. Speak from the heart; honesty is your best business tool.

Don't Let It Ring Twice:
Professional Telephone Skills

How many clients are lost because someone in the salon is too busy to pick up the telephone? I must admit I tend to be an overachiever, so when the salon telephone rings and the receptionist is away from the front counter, I'll answer it in my very best "I'm so glad you called" voice. I have been criticized by fellow salon professionals for what they consider a character flaw. You see, they'd rather let the phone ring than seem over-eager to a client. My response: Be eager.

The telephone is *your* life line to success. It allows you immediate interaction with clients. As with a 60-second decision when you first meet a client, an individual makes a judgment right over the phone line almost instantly when you first speak on the telephone. Because I consider the telephone one of our most valuable resources, allow me to share how to put that next telephone call to work for you.

- ✂ When answering the phone, your voice should be inviting and friendly ("Oh, Katina, it's lovely to talk with you. I'm so glad you called."). Nobody wants to communicate with a sourpuss ("Yea, what do you need?"). Your goal here is to make your voice sound inviting and warm.

- ✂ A smile or a frown is magically transmitted through your voice. People in marketing and sales often keep a mirror on their desks to remind them to smile when talking with clients. People hear a smile in your voice.

- ✂ Turn up your energy level. We've all had tough days. Ask any salon professional, and he or she probably had one just this last week. Even when days are hectic, don't take it out on the next caller. Project your voice as if you were giving a speech or about to sing. To do this, take a good breath, stand or sit tall and speak slightly slower than in normal conversation.

✂ Play with the volume, pitch, and rate as you speak. Change the volume when enthusiastic, go higher or lower and string out words. It's okay to talk in a stage whisper if you're sharing a secret, such as: "Wait till you see it! The salon is being completely renovated (in an excited tone)! It's going to be absolutely "to die for" (in a confidential stage whisper), but of course our prices will remain sensible (down-to-earth tone)." Get the idea? I knew you would.

✂ Talk to your client on the telephone as if the two of you were face to face. Never chew gum, eat or drink when talking on the phone. Try to avoid doing other tasks while talking with clients, such as running the cash register or cutting hair — we've all seen salon professionals balance a phone, and do this type of double duty. The client on the other end of the telephone line knows she or he is not getting full attention and may feel annoyed. Don't you imagine that the client in the chair feels cheated, too?

✂ When picking up the phone, identify yourself immediately. Don't let them guess who is talking. Let's say that Greg, the receptionist, transferred a call to your station. Even though Greg may have said that he'll put you on the phone immediately, it's good business savvy to identify yourself with: "Good morning (afternoon or evening); this is Tony

Smith." The greeting is warm and friendly. It's true that "Hello?" works, but it lacks that professional announcement that you're a confident business person ready to talk with a client. (Stand up when you take a call, and you'll sound even more powerful and poised.)

✂ When you initiate a call, be sure you do so at a convenient time. It's always good manners to ask: "Is this a convenient time to call?" The caller will appreciate your professionalism, and most likely, return it.

✂ Conclude the phone conversation in a timely manner. You can chat with friends when you're home. When in the salon, keep phone calls brief and to the point.

✂ Say "thank you for calling" adding the client's name at the end of the call. You'll leave that person with a warm, inviting feeling.

✂ When taking a message for someone else, be sure to get all the details such as to whom the call is directed, the caller's name, phone number, best time to return the call, and, if appropriate, the message.

✂ The same holds true when leaving a message. Be prepared with the specific items you want to address whether you reach a machine or a person.

When leaving the message, speak slowly, and clearly. Leave your full name (even if you believe the person will immediately recognize your name) and your phone number (and area code if appropriate). Say your name and phone number at a rate you'd appreciate hearing if you were writing it down. Also, always leave your number even if you believe that the person you're calling knows it by heart. Give the time you're calling and a brief indication of the reason for the call.

As my client Bonnie Dean says, she gets so excited when she calls someone, she has to pace herself and always repeats the phone number twice to ensure success.

Use the telephone as a tool. When a client tries a new product or has a special service performed, I always follow up with a phone call. You guessed it. I leave a lot of messages since my clientele is drawn from business people who aren't home during the day. When following up, it's always good to personally interact. However, there are times when I want to tell clients that they need not call me back, and I leave this message, too.

Every time you talk on the telephone, you're holding a resource in your hand that can expand your income, increase your network and add to your professional image. Handle it with care, respect it and boost your business with this practical tool. I always say I'm dialing for dollars. Make every opportunity count.

Thank You: The Note That Counts

When was the last time you thanked your clients for their continuing support of your talents and quality service? No, I'm not talking about a simple, "Hey, thanks, Joy," as the client writes her check. Or, "Appreciate you, Bob," as he hands you a twenty. A sincere "thank you" could be one of your best business tools and the sharpest part of your new professional image. A thank you note written from the heart could very well triple your business next year. That's quite a statement, and it's absolutely true.

With all the anonymity in our high-tech world, those who take time to say a few words of appreciation stand out of the crowd. Those who write a brief note of thanks to their clients are even more of a novelty. They are also the ones who never lack quality clients and are always positive and upbeat about their profession.

Here are some tips to consider as you make your professional presence felt:

- ✂ Send a thank you note to every client, just because. It will take a bundle of time and a roll or two of stamps, but the dividends will be well worth it.

- ✂ Send a brief note of thanks to clients after you provide service. Make them individualized: "That last haircut was really *you!*"

- ✂ Send a client a special note if they've purchased a product that you've recommended. "Hope you love the XX shampoo as much as I do. Your hair did look sensational." You'll cement a sale, and the client will come back to purchase again.

- ✂ If you hear that a client receives a promotion, becomes ill, announces a pregnancy, or is about to retire, dash to the card store during your next break to find a special card for this person.

✂ Keep a record, on your salon cards, of clients' birthdays and organize a birthday book with names, addresses, and dates. When their day is close, send a card. I don't know about you, but the more birthday cards I get, the more special I feel. Making your clients feel valued will keep them loyal.

✂ Haven't heard from a client in a while? Drop him or her a note and follow up with a phone call. People change their minds, and some are afraid to hurt our feelings if a product or service wasn't to their liking. We need to know why and try to help the client solve the problem. It's easier to keep clients than cultivate new ones.

What do you get by taking these steps? Plenty of clients, busy appointment books, and increased income are three of the obvious answers. The one that hits home, however, is that you are considering yourself a professional and going the extra mile to make customer service your key to a better future.

Since we're in the beauty business, it makes sense to look for cards that have to do with beauty. I scan the stores looking for cards that have something to do with hair or beauty. I always buy them up and my clients love them.

Probably one of my most successful thank you's was to my client Marilyn. She constantly sends me new business. So out of the blue I sent her a bouquet of flowers, just to say thank you. The bouquet cost me $25; Marilyn's referral efforts have totaled up to as much as $2,500 in referred business. I'd say that the cost of the flowers was a wise investment.

In Summary

Emily Post, the ultimate authority on etiquette said, "Manners are a sensitive awareness of the feelings of others. If you have that awareness, you have good manners, no matter what fork you use."

As you polish your image, remember:

- ✄ When giving a presentation, be aware of your audience and meet their needs
- ✄ Know that change takes time, and change is usually work
- ✄ Practice excellent telephone skills
- ✄ Say thank you, and share a kind word

You now have the power and the passion, and in the next section, we'll focus on naming and achieving personal and professional goals. *And* we'll talk about how to make more money.

Section 3
Goals:
Making A Mole Hill from That Mountain

By now you know that passion can be yours. Success can be yours. Fulfillment can be yours. They are all achievements of your making if you'll work toward them.

To achieve success and cultivate passion, we must have a plan. Therefore in this very important section, we'll examine goals, how to make them, and how to reach them.

When speaking at seminars on this topic, I've actually overheard salon professionals whisper: "Goals — who needs them? If I work hard, I know I'll get ahead." Is there any credibility to that theory? In one word, no. What you'll end up doing is working very hard and making money, but without a plan (which is a goal), there's every indication that money will be mismanaged. Additionally, without goals time will be squandered and opportunities lost.

When I started out in the business, I held the naive idea that goals were only for stuffy middle-aged folks who didn't have anything better to do than count their spare change. Boy, was I wrong! I'm thankful, though, that I didn't have to learn the necessity of setting goals to achieve success the really hard way. To be truthful before I realized that goal setting was essential, I had lost sight of my objectives for about three years. I realize now that I was fortunate. Some of the people I've talked with don't gain the insight and absolute need for goal setting until it's too late. Quite a few salon professionals fail to make it through the first five years after they graduate from beauty school. They simply drop out and become has beens before they've had a chance. I attribute this failure rate to insufficient goal setting, lack of perseverance, or no goal setting at all.

I can truly say I'm successful. I look back at the years that I've spent in this industry and look at how fortunate I am. By the age of 30, I had reached all of my *lifetime* goals. It was amazing all the things I thought would take years to attain but that I had accomplished. Now I'm setting bigger, more outrageous goals, things I never thought possible. You see the harder I work, the luckier I get.

Juan, who at one time trimmed and snipped the hair of Park Avenue's rich and famous, retired a few years ago at age *45*. Now he facilitates some of the work programs for New York's homeless *and* spends the evenings volunteering his hair-cutting skills at a shelter.

Juan recently told me, "I've been a goal setter since I can remember. You see, when my family moved here from Cuba, we were just lucky to be alive, however I never remember my parents complaining about working. They stressed the satisfaction of work. When I was about ten, I realized that Mama and Dad were not just helping us kids with homework, they were planning our future, budgeting our very limited income, and taking pride in accomplishments. There was always a list of goals taped to the refrigerator door.

"Through the use of goal-setting principles, my parents helped us all through school and on to great career opportunities. Gloria, my baby sister, is an oncologist in Philadelphia; Tina, the oldest, is a clothing designer with a major line, and my brother, Raul, is the best fifth-grade teacher in the Bronx. My parents also planned and invested well for their retirement, and they taught us all to do that. And today? They can afford to be unpaid workers for a refugee organization. Through my own family, I have seen the evolution of the goal-setting process. I've seen two struggling immigrants map a family's future and make that future possible. That's what goal setting did for our family. When I started out in the business, I applied the sample principles and made my successful future a reality, too."

When I was researching and interviewing successful salon professionals for this section, Juan and others pointed out that there is more than one way to set goals. Therefore in this section, you'll have the chance to learn the easiest and most successful formats real people use to get real results. Nonetheless, I'd never ask you to stifle your creativity. You should modify the concepts to work for you, but please do begin setting goals. They work.

Also, in the second portion of this section we'll focus on money. Never have any left? I'll share some information that could change all that. We'll round out the section with some financial planning advice you can start to use today.

Sylvia Porter, the financial whiz and author of *Sylvia Porter's Money Book*, says, "Money can be translated into the beauty of living, a support in misfortune, an education, or future security." Money gives us options so when sketching out your goals, don't hesitate to put *money* on your list.

Set 'Em High: Goals and Achievements

Let's say you wanted to go on a driving vacation this year and travel from the Golden Gate Bridge in San Francisco to the Brooklyn Bridge in New York or vice versa. Without even thinking about traversing more than 3,000 miles, you organize the trip in your head. Various steps would include making sure you had enough vacation time, enough money, and that the car was in good working order. Somewhere in this scheme, you'd plan the route, get other maps (for those great side trips), figure out where you'd stay or camp along the way and wonder what to wear or what snacks to pack.

But what if one afternoon you jumped in the car and got on the first freeway entrance to head out of town. Without a plan, you could get lost, run out of money, or have car problems. Quite a difference when you have a plan, isn't there?

A goal is just a piece of your life plan. Without goals (or these road maps to a better future) you could end up being disappointed and baffled. I believe in goal setting and goal achieving. I believe in having a plan.

Shawn, a business professional in Carlsbad, told me recently that she takes goal setting to the height of luxury. I did a double take since my goal setting usually occurs with a pencil and a yellow tablet, sometimes sitting down with my son as he's working on a school project or finishing homework.

Shawn explained, "Twice a year, I go alone to a wonderful spa on a lake about three hours from the city. It's my goal-setting retreat.

"During the drive, I speculate on what I want to achieve in the next six months, in the next year, five years, ten years and twenty. After a long, contemplative walk in the woods and a gourmet dinner, I get ready for serious goal setting. Sitting on the balcony sipping champagne or in front of the fire with a hot toddy or cocoa — depending on the season — I write my goals. Sometimes they seem more like dreams, but dreams are the basis for all success, aren't they?" Shawn says the alone time is crucial for her thinking process. "My business is really me, and I need to invest time to make it happen."

Is Shawn successful? "I'll be buying my dream house next year." This professional laughs and says that she's about to make goal planning mandatory for her entire staff.

Other salon professionals and successful business people I talked with stress that to make goals work, they must be high enough to challenge us. However, they must be workable enough to be broken down into small, attainable portions.

More so, successful goal-setters give themselves plenty of rewards when they reach their interim and long-term goals. A reward might be something you'll use in your business or a treat that says you're special.

A Self-Evaluated Test for Goal Setters

#1, the *home* test: How do you treat those with whom you live?

#2, the *business* test: How do you conduct yourself toward team members, subordinates, supervisors, and clients?

#3, the *social* test: How do you act toward those who do not enjoy the same social advantages as you? How do you act in social situations when you may not feel comfortable?

#4, the *success* test: How do you behave when favoring circumstances involve wealth, power, position, and honor?

Take the test to heart. Make sure you like your own answers before you begin to renovate others in your life and business.

"If you think you can, you can. And if you think you can't, you're right."
— Mary Kay Ashe

Goals: List Method

The "list method" is one of the simplest forms of goal setting. You write down what you hope to achieve and then on supplemental sheets list the steps necessary to achieve the goals.

The list method has been used with great results by salon professionals (and other dynamic people) throughout the years. Why? Because it works.

On the following pages, you'll find Goal Summary Sheets and Supplemental Summary Sheets to itemize each goal. I've indicated ten places for goals; you may have more. That's great because the more goals the better. Just work up your own extra sheets or photocopy those provided and change the numbers.

Below are examples of a Goal Summary Sheet and Supplemental Sheet to illustrate how to use them. Notice that there's a place for the date and signature on the accompanying worksheets; this is done so that you consider the goals a commitment. This is a contract with yourself to achieve success. Also note that on the Supplemental Sheets there's a "By When" category. Fill this in to indicate when you must begin each step. The completion dates are essential: You must give yourself rules, a starting point and an end date, too. That's why date lines are added on the Supplemental Sheet.

When you finish writing all goals and complete the items on the Supplemental Sheets, place them in an attractive folder or envelope where you can review them often. Some goal achievers post their goal lists in obvious place — top drawer of their desk, on the mirror in the bathroom, etc. They believe that seeing the list helps establish the goals in their minds.

It always amazes me how this works. When I learned the process, I actually took a class and filled out my goals. When I finished the course, I put the notebook away. Six months later, I looked at the notebook and discovered I had attained everything on the list. That was a turning point in my goal setting.

You see, your conscious mind can only go to one thought at a time. But your unconscious mind can do many tasks simultaneously.

Remember: What you think about, you talk about; what you talk about, you bring about.

Goal Summary Sheet

Here are some sample ideas that could possibly be used for a Goal Summary Sheet:

Goal #1: Increase clientele by 50 percent.

Goal #2: Better manage time.

Goal #3: Improve working relations with others in the salon.

Goal #4: Save more money.

Goal #5: Have more time for family/self.

Goal #6: Increase professional flexibility.

Goal Supplemental Sheet

Here is a sample of what a completed Summary Sheet might look like:

Goal #1: Increase clientele by 50 percent. These are the steps I need to take to achieve Goal #1:

	Step	**By When**
1	Become aware of better serving clients	Now
2	Ask for referrals	Now
3	Create referral cards and give them out	4/5
4	Acknowledge clients who make referrals	4/5
5	Talk about my business in business situations	Now
6	Join a networking organization	4/10
7	Join civic or volunteer organizations	5/10
8	Send thank you notes to all clients "just because"	Now
9	Take classes at community college	Fall

Notice in the samples above that the large goal of increasing the client base is divided into small, workable goals. For example, by better serving clients, the person who is formatting the goal list knows that happy clients make recommendations. Actually, they can't wait to tell their friends exactly how wonderful their salon professional is. This is just what needs to be done to increase clientele.

The second step to realizing a larger clientele is to ask for referrals. It sounds so simple, but honestly, when was the last time you did that? Asking for referrals brings in new clients. When your clients are delighted with the professional services you perform, they are proud to help your business. But you must ask for their assistance. I built my whole business with this technique.

In the third step to achieving the first goal, the sample says that referral cards have to be handed out. Referral cards can be fancy or as simple as business cards that have your name and the salon's location and phone. I'd recommend adding a line to acknowledge the person who makes the referral. When the newly referred client comes in, he or she shows you the card so you know exactly who to thank. You can use the card as a reminder to send a note of thanks or follow up with a phone call of appreciation.

Looking at the Goal Summary Sheet once again, it's somewhat daunting to write "Increase clientele by 50 percent" and not know how or when to start. Yet by providing a plan of action with the Goal Supplemental Sheet, it's easy.

Okay, now it's your turn. Use the next few pages to map your own goals. You may want to photocopy the pages and make a few rough drafts or give the extra copies to success-minded colleagues so they can get started on their goals, too.

Goal Summary Sheet

Goal #1:

Goal #2:

Goal #3:

Goal #4:

Goal #5:

Goal #6:

Goal #7:

Goal #8:

Goal #9:

Goal #10:

_____   _____

Signature   Date

Supplemental Summary Sheet

Goal #____: _____

_____

Steps I need to take to achieve Goal #__: By When

1.

2.

3.

4.

5.

6.

7.

8.

9.

10.

Goals: Bubble Method

A growing number of successful salon professionals are also using another system to realize goals. Sometimes called Mind Mapping, I always refer to it as the Bubble Method. It's as fun as it is easy. It's also very effective if you're not sure of the direction you want to take toward success. It works well, too, if you have a knotty decision to make and need a place to visualize your options.

Using the bubble method is very simple. Here's all you have to do:

1. Find a large piece of paper and some colored marking pens or crayons. You'll also want a quiet place to work.

2. In the center of a piece of paper, write a key word that means attainment of your goals. Always print when using the bubble method. You can use the word "success" in the middle. I find it most effective.

3. Draw a circle around the main word.

4. From the circle, draw ten lines in various places around the edge. From each line, print descriptions of how you'll attain success. Then circle each of the ten items.

5. Using ten pieces of paper, print each of the ten items in the center of their own sheet, circle the item and repeat #4. This time, however, further itemize how you will achieve each definition of success.

Some people are able to accomplish all this writing and circling on one sheet of paper. I like to spread out, and I also like to draw and doodle while I'm thinking.

From the sheets, you can then post the final results where you can see your goals and the steps you need to take to achieve them. Or, you can transfer the information to a formal list, as in the List Method.

It doesn't matter which goal-setting method you choose. But it does matter that you write down goals. Keeping them magically encoded in your head might seem more efficient, yet in reality, the mind needs to see them written out to make them happen more easily.

Every year, my friend Tasha gets a group of us together to do goals and goal posters. For goal posters, we cut out pictures and glued them to our goal boards as a visual reminder of what we want. It's a great exercise, and gives us time together with some wonderful food and inspirational company. It also gives us an idea of what each of us wants in life. That way, we can support each other.

"Action is the antidote to despair."
— Joan Baez

Notes On Goal Achieving

✂ Make every plan an action plan.

✂ Plan your work, and work your plan.

✂ Set goals. Only the top ten percent of salon professionals set goals.

✂ Be willing to do whatever it takes to achieve your goals.

✂ Balance your life; make time for you.

Goals: Making A Mole Hill from That Mountain

Insurmountable

It isn't easy

to apologize,

to begin again,

to admit error,

to be unselfish,

to face a sneer,

to be considerate,

to endure success,

to profit by mistakes,

to forgive and forget,

to keep on trying,

to keep out of the rut,

to make the best of a little,

to shoulder deserved blame,

to subdue an ugly temper,

to maintain a high standard,

but it's always worth it.
— Author Unknown

Focus on Business

What do you want from life? How are you going to get it? The needs of the salon professional are considerable. Whether you're working in a salon or own the salon, you are in business. This chapter centers on how to concentrate your goal setting needs and relate them directly to your business.

You may have already guessed that there are no right or wrong answers to the questions below. In the provided spaces, write down your responses to my questions. I have used this questionnaire many times to focus my own business, and I share it with achievers at seminars. Now it's your turn to fill in the blanks and possibly change your life for the better.

Business Description

1. What do you want for your business and yourself? State in general terms.

2. How is your business unique?

3. What are your specific goals? Break them into periods of five years, three years, one year, and six months.

Market Analysis

4. What is the general market you do business in?

5. What is the specific market you have targeted?

6. Who is your competition?

7. What trends in the market and competition can you anticipate?

Products and/or Services

8. What are the product(s) and/or service(s) you offer now or will offer?

9. Who could duplicate these and how?

10. Who are your suppliers?

11. How are you pricing your products and/or services?

12. How do you market and distribute your products and/or services?

Management Plan

13. Who will run your business?

14. How will it be organized and operated?

15. What are the business' strengths and weaknesses?

16. What are the business' opportunities and threats from outside?

Financial Data

17. How much money is available for the business?

18. What is the budget (for Year 1 and quarterly, years 2 - 5 annually)?

19. What is the anticipated income? What's your cash flow?

20. How do you know these numbers are correct?

What do you do now? Review your answers. Are you doing what needs to be done to improve your business? What changes can you make? Review your goals, and write specific goals in these areas. Don't hesitate to talk with successful people in your network for answers; consult with books on business topics, too. You do not need to reinvent the wheel since there is plenty of great business advice available just for the asking.

Finally, and especially if you are puzzled, put the list aside for a few days, and when you review, you'll have a fresh perspective to untangle the most complex knots.

Spending Plan: A Checklist to Check Your Finances

Most of us enjoy spending money. That's a fact of life, yet few people come right out and say it. Many of us in the salon profession love to make money, too. I fit nicely into both categories, thank you very much.

When I first began taking my career seriously, I remember talking with a colleague about spending money faster than I made it. I was frustrated and knew if I couldn't pull myself together on this, I probably wouldn't make it in the business.

Mary had been a salon professional for quite some time and was doing well. She was one of my first role models. Always polite, she listened to me complain, and then asked, "Have you ever written down your sources of income and your expenses?"

"But I've tried a budget..."

"You're missing the point, Susie. All I'm suggesting is that you write down your income, expenses and savings. Write it all out, and keep records. Then you'll stay on target."

Not only did I stay on target, but I could track that target, too.

Here's a plan for you. While your expenses, income sources and ways to save are different than mine, perhaps different than those listed below, use this format as a launching pad to help manage your income.

I also recommend formulating one for your business whether you are the salon owner or an independent contractor with your own business in a salon. Do it in long hand or keep it on your computer, but do it if you're having trouble balancing money with bills.

Financial Checklist

For the month of _____

INCOME SOURCES
Wages or salary:
Bonuses:
Dividends and interest
Child support
Alimony
Rents
Royalties
Fees
Commissions
Tips
Other_____

EXPENSES
Auto expenses (gas, oil, etc.)
Auto loan
Auto repairs and maintenance
Beauty/barber/nail services
Cable TV
Check services
Child care
Church donations
Classes
Clothing
Computer hardware and software
Continuing education
Contributions or tithe
Credit card payments
Doctors and dentists
Entertainment (movies, music, sporting events)
Gambling
Gifts/birthdays/etc.
Groceries
Household expenses
House payment
Income taxes (federal, state, city)
Insurance, auto
Insurance, health
Insurance, home/apartment
Insurance, life
Magazines, newspapers, books
Membership (clubs and organizations)

Personal loans
Property taxes
Retirement plan (IRA or other)
Second mortgage payment
Self improvement
Social security deductions
Sporting equipment
Student loans
Sundries
Telephone (local and long distance)
Textbooks, school supplies
Tobacco/candy
Utilities (gas/electricity/water)
Vacations
Other _____

SAVINGS
Annuities
Certificates of deposit
Savings accounts
Savings bonds
Trust accounts
Other _____

Goals: Making A Mole Hill from That Mountain

Financial Points to Ponder

Point 1: *A plain bar of iron is worth five dollars*

Point 2: *The same bar of iron, when made into horseshoes is worth $10.50.*

Point 3: *If the iron is made into needles, it's worth $4,285.*

Point 4: *If it's turned into balance wheels for watches, it becomes worth $250,000.*

Point 5: *This analogy is true of another commodity ... you. Your value is determined by what you make of yourself.*

Getting a Handle on Money

Now that you know where you stand on your cash flow, you should take this information and do something with it. Take a look at your next possible steps.

- ✄ Talk with a financial planner. He or she can help you format a savings and spending plan.

- ✄ Consult some of the many computer software programs that help people budget and assess their finances. Many programs allow a trial period; if they don't fit your needs, exchange them for others. Ask colleagues what they use and why.

- ✄ Learn to save. If you save a dollar a day, you'll have over three hundred dollars by year's end. That's not a lot, but if you're saving little or none right now, that money will be a good start. Better yet, tithe yourself. That is, put away ten percent of your income before taxes. This works better than you can dream.

- ✄ Refer to the books on financial planning at the bookstore or library. I highly recommend the Consumer Report's book *Our Money, Our Selves*, by Ginita Wall, C.P.A., C.F.P. (Consumer's Union, 1992) to help you manage your money.

- ✄ Consult books on repairing credit if you're in over your head. An excellent book on the topic is *The Consumer's Credit Book: How to Repair or Get Credit*, by Charlene Brown (United Resources Books, 1991).

- ✄ Talk to a company that helps consolidate debts if you're behind in your financial obligations. But enter into agreements with these companies with your eyes open; they charge for their services.

✄ Strive to be in control of your money rather than being controlled by money.

✄ Consider your income as a reward for your hard work.

✄ Learn to cope with your financial responsibilities by keeping bills current. Seek financial freedom by becoming educated. Save for now and for later. Take responsibilities for your own actions. And, protect your credit and reduce financial risk taking.

✄ Realize that money will not end all your problems.

✄ Seek professional counseling if you're having problems with money, including the handling, saving, spending or gambling of it and are out of control.

A solid financial future can begin this very day. The first step is awareness.

Never stop reaching for more:
Do more than exist — live.
Do more than touch — feel.
Do more than look — observe.
Do more than read — absorb.
Do more than hear — listen.
Do more than listen — understand.
— John H. Rhoades

In Summary

Lots of people talk about money being power, but I consider it as a means of providing choices. Money allows us to chart our own professional course in the salon and out. Money helps shape our future. When we budget and set goals, when we plan and recognize our investment challenges, we make choices that not only shape our future but that of our families and extended family of friends.

Ginita Wall, author of books on investments and financial goal setting says, "Your financial future is up to you. No matter what your past financial history has been, you can begin today to build a solid financial foundation." If you've already started building, I urge you to become financially educated so you can reinforce that which you already know.

As you move to the next section, keep these points in mind:

- ✄ Goals make dreams reality
- ✄ Set goals high, yet make them achievable
- ✄ Focus on your business every day
- ✄ Get a handle on money
- ✄ Strive for financial, personal, and professional success

In the next section, we'll address marketing and your role as a salon professional. We're not going to reinvent the wheel. Rather, I'll share some advice that has worked incredibly well for me and others in our industry regarding marketing, selling and managing time.

So if you really want to sky rocket your success with an "E Ticket" to the top of the career ladder, don't skip over any portion of Section 4.

And one more thought to ponder: If you do not think about the future, you cannot have one.

Section 4
Marketing:
Crashing Through to Sales Success

Every professional field has super achievers who seem to know just the right way to market their services, sell their products and network their circle.

In this section, we'll focus on marketing from behind the scenes and reveal these secrets. With this information, you'll begin to work your plan and plan your work through to the finer points of networking for success. There's a lot to learn, and you can immediately incorporate some tips into all of your life in the salon and out.

Remember, great leaders and super-professionals never hoard their knowledge. "The more you give the more you get" is an old adage, but it's never been more true than now in these highly competitive times. Yes, you must know when to give and when to take. With respect to going the extra mile to achieve success, the journey alone can move you from mediocre to miraculous. Now, let's hit the book.

Planning Your Work and Working Your Plan

The title is one adage in which I put a lot of trust. How about you? Do you really have a way to work effectively? What is your plan to make your dreams a reality?

As I said in the last section, in order to achieve your goals, you must break down your objectives into workable pieces. That's your plan. Here are suggestions to help you plan your work, which is important because a sound plan makes marketing easier.

"Sales is not a matter of knowing what you should do — it's a matter of *doing* what you should do. Sales people know everything there is to know; the problems is that they just don't do it," Jeffrey Gitomer, author of *The Sales Bible*.

1. **Planning is a top priority**. You'd never decide to add on a room to your home, to buy lumber, paint and tools, and get to work *without a plan*. Success can't be yours without a plan. Understanding the importance of good planning will help you focus on and achieve your goals.

2. **Get yourself in order**. Establish a regular place and time for planning your plan. Make sure this spot is convenient and comfortable and you can work on your plan with a minimum of disruption. Choose your planning time carefully, too. If you're a morning person, don't make plans to organize at midnight. Utilize the time when you're most productive.

3. **Set aside a regular time for making plans**. Andrea, a salon professional in San Marcos, California, arrives at the salon two or three hours early every Monday morning. Although the salon is open seven days a week, Andrea explains, "Monday is the traditional starting day for the week. That alone puts me in the right frame of mind. Generally, I get into the shop at seven, open the door and

lock it again. I make a cup of tea and work in solitude planning my week, recognizing what goals I want to accomplish, and reviewing my personal and professional needs. I inventory supplies, scan client bookings, and scrutinize the physical appeal of the salon. By the time the other team members come in at nine, I feel like I've got a two-day jump on organization."

4. Set up goals you can accomplish immediately and some that will take determination. If you've skipped over the previous section on various goal-setting methods, take a few minutes to review. They are that important.

Make sure all goals are measurable, attainable and realistic. When setting goals, consider the number of sales dollars you expect to earn, number of products you can show to your clients, the number of new clients, and other activities that specifically involve you and the salon. Always write down your goals.

5. Be practical and realistic. When you're planning your work and working your plan, consider the amount of time you really have for activities. "I originally thought I could put in five extra hours at the salon each week to boost my marketing plan," says Cindy, a nail technician in Vista, California. "This worked great until my baby got sick, the car needed service and my husband changed to the second shift at the station." All was not lost, however, because Cindy recognized that she could do a lot of the marketing — working her plan — from home as long as she used those five hours efficiently.

6. Stick with the plan. It's tempting to give up if you have a set back. Cindy, the salon professional mentioned above, said that she had a few moments when juggling a coughing, feverish toddler and writing thank you notes made the plan seem insane. However, she stuck it out through that first brutal week and realized, perhaps as you have already, that flexibility is the key. She said, "Some days I can only put in ten extra minutes; other days get an hour or two so that I exceed my personal goal."

Make your plan flexible and forgive yourself if you get sidetracked. Get back on with the plan's schedule at the very next opportunity.

7. Think out major changes in your plan before you make them. When setting goals, thoroughly consider what is involved. Because life often travels its own course, you may find that your plan for salon success isn't working as you hoped or is too complicated. Reevaluate your options and think of exercising your options and alternatives before you completely scrap your plan.

8. Periodically evaluate your progress. Keep your plan handy; review it once a week. It feels sensational when you know that your plan is bringing the success you formerly dreamed of achieving. Remember, this is your plan, and if you've formatted it with your needs in mind, it will work for you. Be sure to congratulate yourself when you attain your goals. Cory Clues, whom I met at a seminar, says that when accomplishing any goal, he rewards himself with a treat. Cory explains, "I love music so when I reach a small goal, I buy myself a new CD. A major goal might be to add a new piece of equipment for my stereo system or get tickets to a concert. Any way I do it, I feel great and the reward makes me anxious to accomplish another goal."

9. Talk about your goals and visualize attaining them. From Olympic athletes to super salon professionals, winners visualize their plan and see themselves in the achiever's role. One way is to talk about your desires and how you will manifest them in your life. There is a caution here: Only discuss your goals and visualization of your plans with positive, up-beat people. Let the negative men and women in your life see the results when you achieve your goals.

10. **Know the products you're selling and about the service you offer**. Continually attend workshops, seminars and product demonstrations. Ask for additional sales support or education whenever possible. Become thirsty for knowledge to make what you offer to the client more desirable.

11. **Become familiar with sales and selling practices for your part of the business**. Have all the answers and practice explaining them to clients.

Salon consultant Lauren says, "I rehearse a little presentation about a new product line before telling any of my clients about it. They are great products and I sell bundles. However initially, I didn't know how I would address the fact that I changed from Product X to Product Y after singing the praises of the old product for five straight years."

Lauren told me that she borrowed a giant teddy bear and placed it in a dining room chair. She was trying to pretend she was the salon professional and the bear was a customer. Then she pulled another chair up close, put a brush in her hand and began to explain to "Ted" all the reasons for the change to the new product line. "If anyone saw me — other than my family — I would have been laughed out of the business, but it worked well. I went from selling to a three-foot-tall blue stuffed bear to selling my clients on the new line in an amazingly short amount of time. This dress rehearsal allowed me to do it with confidence."

12. **Offer outstanding service**. In our business, one can't be just okay and be successful. The characteristics are mutually exclusive and cancel out each other. You have to offer superior service from the minute a client calls for an appointment until he or she leaves the salon.

Always be cognizant that the product you really sell is yourself, including your background, experience and know-how. When a client buys from you, he or she trusts your judgment as an expert in the beauty profession. If you fall short of superior, you will lose your clients' faith in you.

13. **Share your enthusiasm**. Maintain a positive attitude while planning your work and working your plan. Your outlook should radiate the success you are determined to achieve. Your enthusiasm will then be reflected in the services you perform and the products you sell.

14. **Be progressive and move with the shakers of our occupation**. Educate yourself on the newest products and tools and if possible incorporate them into your working life. Use other high-tech tools to make your business run like a business, including a personal computer, voice mail, car phone, pager, and support staff. Take yourself seriously as a salon professional and others will take you seriously, too. As singer Kenny Rogers says, "Don't be afraid to give up the good to go for the great."

Winners' Words to Remember:

1. *The five most important words: "I am proud of you."*

2. *The four most important words: "What is your opinion?"*

3. *The three most important words: "If you please."*

4. *The two most important words: "Thank you."*

5. *The smallest word of all: "I."*

Defining Your Plan

It's that time...time to define your success plan. By clarifying your plan, you take the first steps in producing a marketing plan. Go slowly because if you miss any of them, you'll miss out on a portion of success that could boost your income into the top 10 percent of the industry.

Vince Pesce, author of *A Complete Manual of Professional Selling: The Modular Approach to Sales Success,* says to improve your planning, take these steps.

1. Identify the areas in your career that need better planning.

2. Identify where you feel dissatisfied with previous performance.

3. List the areas in order of priority.

4. Set a timetable for their improvement.

5. Define the positive action to be taken to accomplish the change.

Sales Savvy

No matter what you sell, where you sell it, or what you do in the salon, a sale in which you're involved can be broken down into the following stages: Qualifying, interviewing, presenting, and closing. Are you rushing any of these? If you hesitated even for an instant, the answer is probably yes.

Most salon professionals wouldn't be caught dead being referred to as a sales person. The truth is we are selling all of the time. I'm selling my clients on why they want to return. I'm selling my kids on what to eat. I'm selling my husband, Bert, on why we're going on vacation. It's a natural process.

So you need to be clear that what we sell are good feelings and solutions. By creating more solutions for our clients and looking for the service you can provide, you have supported them.

Let's examine each stage and find solutions to boost sales and client satisfaction with the services you provide.

Qualifying: This is also called prospecting or cold calling, and we do this the first time we introduce a product to a new client. We do this when we're consulting on what's best for the client and how we can help the client achieve his or her grooming goals. At this stage, we ask questions like: What challenges do you have with your hair? When did you like your hair (nails or skin) the most? Allow your clients to share their hair (nail or skin) challenges. Each challenge is an opportunity to *solve* and provide a service.

Interviewing: In this process you create trust and credibility. Clients may have fears and may need your assurance that you are a professional and confident about the result of the service you provide. This process is the key to winning the client.

In the interviewing process, we discuss the past, present and future with the client regarding the use of products or services. In the interviewing phase, you discover special problems and concerns. You ask for details of past experiences with products or services and what the client hopes to achieve. It is at this time you want to learn pertinent facts about your client to help you market your services or products in the most effective way.

Presenting: This is one of the favorite phases of sales and marketing for many in the industry. We love new products, the smell, the smoothness and the profit. Yet in the presentation stage we must show the client how the product or service solves the problems identified in the interview stage.

For example, let's say that Tina, a new client, loves to swim but suffers from very dry hair that has been permed and colored at home. She readily admits that she has created a hair-care nightmare. You have a new product especially for over-processed hair. It's a conditioner that can't be beat. In this phase, you'd draw attention to that feature and might say that by using it, along with wearing a swim cap while swimming and a sun hat when gardening, it will help restore her hair to a natural beauty. You may also stress the length of time it will take to restore the hair to a healthier condition and various other treatments, including a cut or shaping that will expedite the desired result. Also, you might say, "Tina, it's my recommendation..." This way you are creating a professional image and position. You are giving choices to your clients.

Your goal in this stage of sales is to appeal to something with which the client can identify. In the above example, the client knows the salon professional cares because there is a plan to solve the hair trauma.

Closing: Ask for the sale. Lots of salon professionals fall short on this because they simply don't ask. Let's face it. Nobody likes the word "no." If they say, "I'm using XYZ on your hair. Doesn't it feel luscious (or smell good, etc.)? It's $10.95 here in the salon. Is there any reason why you wouldn't like to take this home?" And if you don't ask? You'll never know if you have completely served the client. I always teach my kids that ASK equals GET. When you ask you get a response, you don't have to ponder or wonder. After a while, you realize that "no" means "no" and nothing more. It doesn't mean you are a bad person or your service was not great. If you have to assign meaning to it, try this. You should have given more information. Something was obviously unclear to the customer.

In the salon, it's possible to proceed through all four phases with one appointment. It's also possible that it could take you months or even years of appointments to go from that initial phase to a sale. It all depends on how you present the product or services you offer. It may also hinge on other items such as the economy, the atmosphere in the salon and your attitude toward the client.

At any given point in this sales savvy cycle, your objective is to move from where you are to the next stage. In other words, if you are in the qualifying phase, move to the interviewing. If you are interviewing, proceed to the point where your client is comfortable with the presentation and continue from there.

Keep this rule in mind: Move from one stage to the next when the client is ready to do so, and don't skip a stage.

Some salon professionals see their work as only one stage, the closing stage. They immediately talk about the product or service and then ask for an answer. It's a wonder they get any "Yes" responses at all. They fail to realize the cyclical nature of sales and by rushing the sale, they lose it.

Let's move out of the salon and into the vegetable garden for a quick analogy. Let's say you decide to plant a garden. One morning you walk outside to perfectly prepared soil and sow seeds for tomatoes. If you're a smart gardener, you realize that it's going to take most of the summer for the tomatoes to progress from the seed stage to your salad bowl. If you pluck the seedlings emerging from the soil, you won't have tomatoes worth eating. But the patient gardener who allows the tomato plants the time needed to mature, eventually harvests juicy, red tomatoes. If the process is rushed, the results will be meager or non-existent.

Selling is like gardening. There are certain things that take time to nurture. Otherwise, you might find that you're not selling, but turning into a professional collector of salon client rejections.

According to sales and marketing experts, we shouldn't attempt a sale the minute we shake hands with a client. This is rushing through the stages. The experts state that it's actually disastrous and could have severe repercussions on our business since we'll be known as a person who is too aggressive.

Most of us are less obvious than sitting a client down and immediately trying to sell a product or service. Yet, many salon professionals never get to the presentation stage, they want to rush the sale. Why? I think it has more to do with trying to please the client than anything else. If we're selling a product or service, we know (or should know) that we're offering quality. We really want the client to know it. Yet, people accept at various speeds so if a client isn't ready for a presentation or for the close, avoid rushing. Make a suggestion, i.e., "Here's a sample of gel. Take it home and let me know how you like it."

The sale wasn't closed, but it wasn't lost either. Your next step will be to include the same query in the thank you note you always send after a client visits the salon. In the note you'll want to add a postscript of: "How did you like that gel? Shall I save a bottle for you?" Then put a reminder on the client's card to ask again during the next appointment. Of course, if he or she says it wasn't desirable, you can easily go back to the interview stage.

We are in the salon to solve problems and help. That's the role of sales, too.

> *"I don't know the key to success, but the key to failure is trying to please everybody."*
> — Bill Cosby

Top Points in Selling

1. *Sell yourself on the fact that you can sell.*
2. *Don't make selling hard because it's not.*
3. *Take the positive approach.*
4. *Have faith:*
   ...in God
   ...in yourself
   ...in your product
   ...in your customer
5. *Know that the right word at the right time can make a sale.*
6. *Be punctual and follow through.*

Retail Equals Retention

Retailing is an absolute must for salon professionals. Yet, for some bizarre reason, many of us ignore or neglect this aspect of assisting our clients and promoting ourselves and our careers.

Before you shake your head and argue that retail "isn't my cup of tea," give me a moment to explain this money-making analogy.

You're with a new client. He or she is very satisfied with the services you provide and you seem to have a good business relationship. But, as we both know, with "first-timers" there is always the chance that they won't return. What's a salon professional supposed to do?

First, let's see what marketing and retailing experts say happens if the clients buys a retail product. If this client purchases one product, there's a 30 percent chance that he or she will return. If a client purchases two products, that figure is increased to 60 percent. And if they purchase three products from you, there's a 90 percent chance that he or she will return for more services.

This isn't about hard or soft selling. It's about client retention. Many salon professionals falsely believe, "Yuck! The owners just wants me to hawk these products." Not true. Typically retail isn't about that at all; it's about really servicing your clients. It's about finding the need and filling the need. It's about being a business entrepreneur.

Along with the aspect of providing answers, retailing allows us to supply education to our clients in order to retain them. The commercials on television for beauty products are not going to educate our clients nor will the ads in the glossy magazines. It's up to us to help clients with their grooming and beauty concerns and fulfill their desires.

As you know, many consumers do not fully understand the distinction between salon products and those sold at the grocery store. As professionals in the industry, we must show clients the differences between the products; we cannot nor should not attempt to make their decisions. It is our job to help them understand exactly why salon products are better, more concentrated, better quality ingredients, etc. Additionally, we need to explain that some of the revenue generated by the sale of salon products helps salon professionals in their careers and endeavors. Clients will not begrudge you for furthering your career as you explain that the sale of the products helps you learn more so you can give more service back to that client and others who visit your salon.

If we can identify the clients' needs, say with a detangler or a sculpting lotion, we can then fill a real need. If we take that perspective, rather than "I've got to sell," we do two things. First, we increase our revenues (most salon professionals earn from 10 to 20 percent on retail items) and second, we build trust.

Through educating, identifying and filling the need, a rewarding connection is established. I know it goes even a step further since clients purchase because they feel the salon professional cares enough to discuss how they can look their best. Isn't it gratifying when a client comes back and says, "Gee, that shampoo (or spray or whatever) was wonderful. My hair has never been better"? This is the way we're really able to give a client something no one else can give. By doing so, clients will stay right there where they belong — on our client list.

By understanding your special relationship with clients and the service you perform through education and as you satisfy their needs, you discover your unique selling philosophy. That's what we'll discuss next. If you have not yet discovered yours, you're not serving your clients as well as you could.

Unique Selling Philosophy

What's so unique about selling? How can it have its own philosophy? Simple. Selling is unique in its philosophy because you are unique. You are special. No one will handle a sale, whether it's a service or a product, exactly like you.

Let's say you're a hair designer. What do you have to offer me that any other designer doesn't? Maybe a lot of experience. But so what? Other people in the salon probably have that much experience...or more. Maybe you have more clients than any other professional in the salon. Again, so what? The client doesn't really care.

How are you different, unique from your competitor? Think how you begin your day. Do you go into the salon with a positive attitude? Is your area sparkling and inviting? Do you greet everyone with a smile, handshake, and upbeat conversation? Are you prompt and courteous? If you're running late or handling an emergency, do you give your clients options and/or honestly tell them how long you'll be tied up? Do you leave every client with a hug or touch, and put a thank-you note in the mail the same day you've provided a service? Do you look for ways to help solve a client's beauty concerns and grooming or fashion questions? Do you try to give guidance and assistance even before the questions are asked? By putting your client first, you will stand ahead of the competition.

Let's examine the relationship between you and your client. Do you educate as you go? For example, when you're selecting a shampoo, do you explain why you've chosen Brand X over Brand Y? When you use a polish remover or a color or a perm, explain why you've arrived at the decision so your client accepts you as an expert. He or she will understand that you truly care because you've used a shampoo for fine hair or a color that works best with gray hair, etc.

In other words, don't keep your clients in the dark. Let them know you care about them because of the choices you are making and the product that you are using.

I challenge you to identify your uniqueness and educate your clients by using the above information for the betterment of your business. You needn't discount those qualities of customer satisfaction that work — just incorporate them into your special style. Do it today.

To become an expert in your field, whether you are a color expert, natural nail technician or perm specialist, decide on your niche and capitalize on it. Many of us wander aimlessly trying to be all things. For instance, I want every client to depend on me for regular chemical services, so I've worked to attract clients who need to see me every four to six weeks for those services. I am guaranteed a salary I can count on and money to put in the bank by achieving this goal and by discovering my niche, I have discovered my uniqueness. I believe that if you don't stand for something, you'll fall for anything.

Ten Commandments of Superior Customer Service and Retention

CLIENTS are the most important people in any business.

CLIENTS are not dependent on us; we are dependent on them.

CLIENTS are not an interruption of our work. They are the purpose of it.

CLIENTS do us a favor when they call on us. We are not doing one by serving them.

CLIENTS are part of our business, not outsiders.

CLIENTS are human beings, like ourselves, with the same feelings and emotions.

CLIENTS bring us their needs. It is our job to satisfy those needs.

CLIENTS are not those to argue or match wits with.

CLIENTS are deserving of the most courteous and attentive treatment we can give them.

CLIENTS are the life blood of our business and every other business.

Client Retention

Do you know that if you continue to build your business and attract new clients while retaining *just* 5 percent of your regular clients throughout a one-year period, your profits will rise more than 25 percent? Can you imagine what that percentage would be if you retained 10 percent of your regular clients? How about 80 percent? It's easier to keep one client, marketing experts state, than to attract five new ones.

Do you know that disgruntled clients — regardless of their reason — will go out and tell seven other people about what went wrong with their last visit to your salon. Can we really afford to lose clients? The obvious answer should make you ponder ways to retain your clientele.

The bottom line? The client skills you display will attract, keep or reject clients.

Marketing Practices That You Need

Since the first salon professional said, "Here, try this sample," we've been searching for ways to market our services and products. Some are subtle and some are in the clients' faces. Here are the best marketing tactics I've used and shared. Take and use those you want, put the others aside for the time being, but don't discount any of the techniques. It's not one thing we do, but all the things. It's better to do a little of everything and distribute your time, than to put all your efforts into one project.

Salon Strategies That Work for You

✂ Salon ploys can snag a client's attention, but once that attention has been snagged, it's up to you to pull through the sale.

✂ Ask for the order once you get the client's attention.

✂ Ask for the sale in terms that your client can understand and stress what you or the product can do.

✂ Think of money as a gimmick. When people receive money they feel obligated to say yes. You might want to put a crisp dollar bill in with your "welcome to the salon" note — or even design "salon money," which is actually a discount coupon for service over a certain amount.

✂ Format a clever way to introduce yourself. Not only does this gimmick help people know you immediately, but they remember you longer, too. For example, I sometimes introduce myself as Susie the Stylist. If I'm feeling flashy, I might say: Susie the Sophisticated Stylist, or Susie the Smashing Stylist.

✂ Give awards in and out of the salon. As an example, you might donate money as a scholarship to a qualified high school student who is going to enter the beauty industry.

Advertise Where It Counts

- ✂ If you're advertising in the Yellow Pages, put the bulk of your advertising dollars there.

- ✂ When preparing an ad or marketing campaign, convey that you are the best in the business. This is no time to feel insecure or shy.

- ✂ Set up a creative team. Hire a freelancer who works for an ad agency; contact the local community college or art school for others on your team. Use young, fresh talent to help design your ads (you'll probably be able to barter services and/or have new clients, too).

- ✂ Think outrageously. Make an scandalous offer to get new clients in the door.

- ✂ Write an advertorial to tell newspaper and magazine readers about you and your specific talents. Offer your services to write a weekly column in your hometown newspaper.

- ✂ Help clients find you. Make your ad or marketing campaign so clear that your phone number jumps right off the page. Don't make clients search for you.

- ✂ Spread the word that you want new clients by asking regular clients to tell others. Clients are not psychic, but they really feel great when they can give the help you ask for.

- ✂ Determine your advertising budget and stay within the guidelines.

- ✂ Barter services to stretch your ad dollars.

✄ Consistency is the key. Stick to your marketing plan. Experts claim that a client has to see an ad ten times before he or she takes action. Be patient and your rewards will be grand.

Get Noticed

✄ Volunteer with local charities, but don't give away your services just because. Have a goal or desired outcome.

One year our salon volunteered our services at a local playhouse and did all the wigs for the plays. I didn't have any idea what I was in for; it was a lot of work. For our involvement, the playhouse management gave us free advertising in the theater programs. Our salon name was seen by nearly five thousand people in the community. That was well worth all the energy.

✄ Become active in a professional network. Get on a committee and do your hardest to make the committee look great.

✄ Don't wait patiently to fill a chair seat on a committee, offer to fill it.

✄ Sponsor an event to help your community.

Two years ago, I organized a fund raiser for Patty. She had a rare skin disease that resulted in her fingers and legs having to be amputated. Patty is a vivacious and outgoing woman and a joy to be around. We had a cut-a-thon/nail-a-thon on her behalf. I enrolled distributors and salon professionals to donate their time to support Patty.

The event was televised by the local cable company and a major television station. All told, we raised $6000 for the day in haircuts and another $10,000 in donations. The community involvement was amazing. It was probably one of the most rewarding events I have ever been involved with.

The happy ending is that Patty is doing extremely well now. Her outlook on life is amazing. Patty doesn't see her disability as a handicap, but just a challenge. She's an inspiration to all of us.

✄ Create a publicity stunt for charity — the more off beat the better.

✄ Don't keep your good work a secret. Write press releases and send them to the local media.

✄ Take a media representative out to lunch. Start building a relationship to get local coverage for your business and other gimmicks you'll do for marketing.

Position Yourself

✄ Forget the thought that if you work hard, you'll be noticed for your high standards. Nonsense. Let people know you're out there working hard and they'll flock to your business.

✄ People hire people. Be the person that people want to hire.

✄ You're always on stage. You are your business. Never forget that people are looking at you as a role model for the need you fill.

✄ Let the world know you're a business professional; carry your business cards everywhere. Hand them out; they don't do any good sitting in your pocket or purse.

Rebbecca, one of my mentors, shared this strategy: Give out five cards a day. That's 25 a week, 100 a month. Make it a goal and your business cards will start paying for themselves.

Remember, consistency and persistence pay off.

✂ Keep abreast of what's innovative in your field.

✂ Give each client some exciting news.

✂ Discover your uniqueness and use it.

Promoting Yourself and Your Company

Do you want to create new interest in yourself and/or your salon? Do you want to add credibility, enhance your image, and bring in new business? Then an excellent promotional plan is just what you need.

Here are some tips from super promoters:

1. **Use contests**. Design a contest where you have a lot of winners and let your clients know how they can win. I often hold contests at the salon for those clients who provide the most referrals during a specific period. Prizes include a gift certificate at a department store or a special restaurant or for services in my salon.

Colleen, a salon professional specializing in kids cuts in the Charlotte, North Carolina area, held a coloring contest for her young clientele. Prizes included coloring books, ice cream cones and a gift certificate at a toy store. Tad Summerset, in the Fort Worth area, sponsored a pie-eating contest at the local fair with the winners getting everything from one haircut to a bundle of hair-care products especially for the men who frequent his busy barber shop.

These may not be the most unique ideas, but they still work. Put on your thinking cap and create something fun and get publicity through a contest. Be sure to tell the media, too.

2. **Write a newsletter and send it to your clients and prospective clients**. Some advertising and publishing companies provide ready-to-photocopy formats of newsletters. I recently enjoyed one from my local printer because it had wonderfully refreshing jokes and human interest anecdotes, like those from *Reader's Digest*. Use your personal computer with a newsletter software program to work it up, or hire a student at the local technical college to create the newsletter for you. When sending your newsletter, make sure you include everyone on your team (and your extended network) in the mailing. Your dentist, the cleaner, alumni association and the store where you buy that fabulous coffee should be on your list. These people are wonderful sources for clients and referrals.

3. **In newsletters or advertisements, include coupons for services**. For example, you might include a gift with purchase, or a free deep conditioning with every perm, or work out an arrangement with the salon's nail technician for a free mini manicure with every coloring. You'll both get new clients.

4. **Put on seminars**. You can offer your specialized services to other salon professionals or to the public. Be sure to charge so your seminar is deemed to be more valuable. Schedule the event at a convenient time for the participants you want as new clients. After the seminar, follow

up with phone calls and/or thank-you notes (possibly adding a discount for future services).

With a salon in San Diego, Sonni puts on make up and hair care seminars for service associations and the public. Sonni has had so much response from business leaders and professionals, that reservations are now required. Included in the price of the seminar, participants try out various hairstyles with the computerized styling programs, learn the latest make up tips and fashion news. They may also pay a little extra for a mini-make over.

5. **Donate your services.** Never feel forced to give your services for free, but do make donations of your services. For example, one evening a month staff members at a salon in Spokane visit nursing homes, a crisis center for women and children, and a Veteran's Administration Hospital giving free haircuts to residents. The publicity from this self-less act has generated many wonderful clients who hear about the work through the coverage given by the local television news. More so, the work makes the staff feel great. There's another side, too, because the donation of services gives the staff plenty of positive reinforcement with established clients.

6. **Give samples.** Everyone loves to test new products and they'll remember your graciousness. But remember to follow up the next time they come in.

7. **Give bonuses and benefits to your clients.** Everyone knows about frequent flier discounts — what about a frequent cutter or color bonus?

8. **Make it special with some specials.** Grocery stores and department stores schedule sales. It's time you thought of this promotion too.

Let clients know when you're having any type of "special." For instance, September might be "Hair Coloring Month," December might be "Holiday Hair Month," and during March you could hold a "Spring Perm Extravaganza." During these sale periods (advertised in your newsletter, fliers, or local paper), promote the discounts for services.

A Sure-Fire Promotion

On the next page, you'll find a promotional planner I've used with great success. It's a list that is so simple you can't go wrong. For ideas on how to promote, review this section and especially the chapter called "Marketing Practices That You Need," or talk with colleagues who have been successful with marketing promotions.

The only "rule" is that you plan one promotion each month; in doing so, you write it with the action steps and follow through. This is your plan and you must work your plan to make it a success.

Be sure to photocopy the plan so that you are working from the copies. You'll need at least twelve copies to organize your year-long marketing program.

Promotional Planner

My promotion for the month of _____

My promotion is: _____

_____

_____

_____

_____

_____

Action steps I need to create my success:

1.

2.

3.

4.

5.

6.

7.

8.

9.

10.

Leadership and Followship: Seven Characteristics

1. *A follower says, "Nobody knows." A leader says, "Let's find out."*

2. *A follower makes a mistake and says, "It wasn't my fault." A leader makes a mistake and says, "I was wrong."*

3. *A follower goes around a problem, but never gets past it. A leader goes through it.*

4. *A follower makes promises. A leader makes commitments.*

5. *A follower says, "I'm not as bad as a lot of other people." A leader says, "I'm good, but not as good as I ought to be."*

6. *A follower tries to tear down those who are superior. A leader tries to learn from those who are superior.*

7. *A follower says, "That's the way it's always been done." A leader says, "There ought to be a better way to do it."*

The Ultimate Test of Time

Time is everywhere and it's nowhere. It's here today and oops, it's gone.

Here's a quick test to check your attitudes toward time and its management. Circle all the answers that are *most* like you. Be honest and you'll get plenty of honest insight.

Y   N   1.   I am occasionally late for meetings and appointments.

Y   N   2.   I sometimes stay late at work when I'd rather be home.

Y   N   3.   Some days, I feel I've accomplished very little of what I wanted to do.

Y   N   4.   I think a problem should be pondered over a period of time before a decision can be made, especially if it's an important concern.

Y   N   5.   I am occasionally suspicious of those who seem to glide through their day without any hassle and who leave the salon and are still smiling.

Y   N   6.   I skip lunch and don't take breaks to keep up with my work.

Y   N   7.   I find it difficult to cope with mistakes made by others in the salon.

Y   N   8.   The balance I have in my savings account is less than I planned to have one year ago.

Y   N   9.   I think of myself as a perfectionist.

Y   N   10. My work day's pace fluctuates drastically.

In reviewing this quiz, you may be shocked to know that time management gurus say that all your answers should have been no. If you answered yes, it means that there may be areas of your work life that need to be organized.

Tests like these don't provide all the answers, yet they're used to heighten awareness that time — a valuable component of success — must be used wisely. Let's see the ways in which you can streamline your day and ensure productivity as we investigate time management.

Do It, Delegate It, or Dump It:
A Jolt in Time Management

Since the beginning of the section, we've focused on client needs, marketing and sales. Now let's look at an aspect of sales people forget: Time management. If you're unable to use time effectively, not only will your clients be unhappy but you'll lose money. And that's the bottom line. If you skipped the quicky quiz above, you may want to return to it. It helps to focus you on the thinking process involved with time management.

To be successful, we must improve and sharpen time management and organizational skills. Not all of us were born with this faculty encoded in our minds; most salon professionals are not clock watchers. Often time gets away from us, and like money pouring through our fingers, we lose sight of our goals. Sometimes we make clients angry when they have to wait too long.

Peggy Sue, a salon owner in California, heard me speak on goals and time management and stayed after the crowd went on to another presentation. Peggy Sue explained that during my presentation, she "felt like you were talking just to me, rather than the entire audience. I'm one of those people who is chronically late and you're absolutely right — I lose clients and the receptionist is constantly upset with me. I know you're writing a book, Susie, so will you please include enough information on time management so that other salon professionals don't have to travel the bumpy road I've just been on."

When asked if Peggy Sue was going to use the information offered to help solve her time management problems, she pursed her lips and said, "Until today, I thought I might have to get out of the business. You can't imagine how much you've done for me — to get me thinking. I can see at least 20 ways to make my business work and it all comes down to effective time management."

As I've found out traveling the country and talking with people in our business, time management is one of the least discussed, but most crucial, components of success. For all the Peggy Sue's, Jimmy's, Jack's and Ginny's out there who are having trouble with the effective use of time, here are some tricks and tips I swear by.

1. **Evaluate your schedule**. Do it ruthlessly and be honest. As you're looking over your daily schedule, review the amounts of time you allow for your business, your personal life, and for you personally.

2. **Review your goals**. If you have yet to formalize them, return to Section 3 and set up goals to help in your business. Reviewing your goals, ask yourself if they are working for you. Make sure you can answer yes.

3. **Write a list of your personal and professional priorities**. I like to keep three lists: *Things To Do, Things I'd Like To Do* and *Optional Things That Would Be Nice to*

129

Do. For example, on the first list I might include "refurbish shampooing area" or "restock supplies," such as thank-you notes and birthday cards. The second list might include: "Attend two networking meetings this week," or "Buy new tapes on sales and motivation." The third list could include: "Have a facial," "Get the car washed and waxed," or "Connect with business associates to exchange ideas."

4. **Plan your time**. Make a list for each day of the six most important things that you need to do that day. This is the real basis for time management. If you don't plan what you want to accomplish, you won't accomplish what you've planned. Or to think of this in another way, if you keep doing what you've always done, you're going to keep on getting what you've always gotten. Are you really satisfied?

5. **Prioritize every item on your list**. Don't overwhelm yourself.

6. **Select what you want to accomplish and do it**. Allow time in your career for doing business that's not strictly interfacing with clients. For instance, you need time for consultation meetings, follow-up time with prospective clients, follow-up phone calls with clients, booking appointments, deliveries, research, and running errands for your business. When you're running errands, carry note paper, post cards, pen and stamps. Whether you're stuck in gridlock traffic or waiting to see the dentist, use this "extra" time to organize and write notes.

7. **Remind yourself that you are valuable**. At the end of each work week, review your schedules and your "Things" lists. Did you reach your daily and weekly goals? After reviewing the lists, make up your list for the next week. Initially, this may sound like a weighty process, but

within two weeks, a time manager may be discovered within you.

8. **Conduct your business like a business.** It's not easy to stay focused as an independent contractor or salon owner. Because you are responsible for your own actions and success, take responsibility seriously and become your own boss. So, organize all supplies that you need for serious work, dress in an appropriate manner to remind yourself that you are doing business (not going out for a date), and teach your family and friends to respect your business hours.

Birmingham resident David, a salon professional with whom I network, told me how he had serious time-eating problems. As a cello player with a classical jazz group, David was encountering chaos in his two careers. Musicians and booking agents called the salon, since they knew David would be there. Of course, he'd get calls from clients, too. Actually the telephone was never quiet with David getting so many calls. And David? He never seemed to have enough time to return all the calls.

Maybe you've recently received phone calls at the wrong time or seen it happen to another team member in the salon. You know the scenario. David would be adding the final snips to an exacting hair cut, and someone would call. The receptionist would put the caller on hold, interrupt David, break into the relationship with the client, be told to take a message *and* then David could get back to work. David is great with customer service — going more than the extra mile — so clients never felt cheated, but David said he was going nuts as he tried to please fellow musicians, agents, clients, and himself.

"One afternoon as I swallowed an aspirin, I looked at the furrows in my forehead and said 'hold the phone.' I meant it literally. I now have voice mail for my musical life, returning those calls before leaving the salon. Clients' calls are returned on the hour; just knowing I'll return their calls satisfies them." Clients now have a relaxed David all to themselves; musicians and agents can leave messages. "And I have more time. One little bit of time management worked a miracle, but I just marvel at what a mess I'd made of life before."

9. **Hold the phone**. As David found out, taking any calls when one is working can be a major time waster. Ask clients, friends, family, and significant others to leave messages. They will if they know you'll be reliable about returning the calls. Be aware of how much time you're actually spending on the phone. Don't forget your friends and loved ones, but when you're in the business arena, restrict your calls to those about business.

10. **Keeping track of your business income is essential not only at tax-paying times, but also for your peace of mind**. Maintain separate checking accounts for business and personal life. Don't mingle your funds. Software programs for your personal computer can help organize your business and personal finances, so make a habit of using them.

11. **Organize your business area and your client files**. Keep them up to date.

12. **If you're not doing something in your business life that is essential, review time management rules and then** *do it*. If there's something that conflicts with your time, *delegate it*. Or, if the issue or problem or chore simply doesn't matter, *dump it*. Don't let issues and items

hang over your head. Remember: **do it, delegate it, or dump it**.

I recently got a call from Peggy Sue, the salon professional who was about to leave the field because she couldn't keep time on her side. The great news is that her business is beginning to thrive. "You'll love this," she told me. "Now other people in the salon are coming to *me* for advice. The receptionist asked if I could help organize her area and the salon owner wants me to mentor two new staff members on the topic of time management. What a kick!"

"Hard work is an accumulation of easy things that should have been done last week."
— Kathy Griffith

Booking Strategies

Do you: Want to make more money every day? Want to see more clients? Here's a booking strategy that works for me and not only keeps things rolling more smoothly, but also keeps me more focused on my work.

Do you take appointments on the hour? Most of us in the business do. However if you make appointments on the half hour or 45 minutes, you'll increase your income.

For instance, let's say you're doing chemical work such as a perm. Why can't you balance the chemical work between hair cuts? Let's say you've booked a perm for eight in the morning. It generally takes 30 minutes to wrap and 20 minutes to process a perm. Within this window of 20 minutes, you have an incredible opportunity to boost your productivity and increase your income. There's no reason why you cannot do a haircut in the extra 20 minutes.

Let's examine this more closely. If a client is receiving a hair coloring, it takes about 15 minutes to formulate, mix, and apply. The color needs 35 to 45 minutes to process. Why not be more productive and use that 35 to 45 minutes to make more money rather than to read a magazine?

It's interesting to see how we use time for our tasks and routines in the salon. For instance, have you ever set a timer to see how long it takes you to do a weave or wrap a perm? Could you be more productive?

My philosophy is simple: I move my hands as fast as my mouth. Check yourself and see how many times you stop and how many times you are not being as productive as you could be.

In strict dollars and cents terms, effectively using extra time is like suddenly giving yourself a raise. Would you ever turn down a raise? What a crazy question. Then try this technique and you'll have more money in your wallet and bank account. This technique alone could earn you hundreds of dollars.

Sure it takes some juggling and often the assistance of someone else in the salon. I had a recent beauty school graduate help me — and of course she was paid. But more so, she learned to balance her time, book on the half hour and the techniques I've used in the salon for years. This young woman is excited about the profession and knows how to use many of the time-management skills discussed within these pages.

With an intern program, you can have students assist you and learn from you. It's a wonderful plan. Call the

Cosmetology Coalition or the Cosmetology Association in your town for more details.

I encourage you to book tighter and make the most effective use of every minute you're in the salon. Like any new time management system, you may feel slightly off kilter at first. I promise that you'll look back and wonder why in the world you wasted so much time in the "between" times.

Working Smart

Motivational master Dale Carnegie once told the story of two men who were out chopping wood. One man worked hard all day, took no breaks, and only stopped briefly for lunch. The other chopper took several breaks during the day and a short nap at lunch. At the end of the day, the woodman who had taken no breaks was quite disturbed to see that the other chopper had cut more wood than he had.

He snapped, "I don't understand. Every time I looked around, you were sitting down, yet you cut more wood than I did."

His companion asked, "Did you happen to notice that while I was sitting down, I was sharpening my ax?"

The moral? Use your time wisely. It's the only time you have and when it's gone, it's gone forever.

Making Time

If from the very instant you awaken until you go to sleep, your time is committed and if you simply cannot find the time to do the things you'd like, here's how to make time.

- ✂ Delegate house work or housekeeping chores.

- ✂ Eliminate some of the work entirely.

- ✂ Make sure everyone at home and in the salon has responsibilities. Make sure you praise the completion of the chores — positive reinforcement breeds more positive behavior.

- ✂ Use small bits of time efficiently.

- ✂ Carefully plan leisure time. It's too easy to get trapped into activities that use time, but give no real pleasure. Don't waste time on unwanted activities.

- ✂ Don't cram your personal appointment book with things to do. Leave some open-ended time for spontaneous activities, to do some mental reorganization, or to meditate.

Some Salon Professionals Are...

A lot of salon professionals are like wheelbarrows,

no good unless they are pushed.

Some are like kites. If a string isn't kept on them,

they fly away.

Some are like kittens.

They are more contented when petted.

Some are like balloons,

full of wind and ready to blow up.

Some are like footballs.

You can't tell which way they'll bounce next.

Some are like trailers.

They have to be pulled.

Some are like lights.

They keep going on and on.

Many thank goodness, are like the North Star.

They are there when needed, dependable, and ever loyal

and a guide to all people.

In Summary

This section has centered on how to really turn your business into a five-star success by cashing in on the marketing and sales possibilities that are all around.

As you move to the next section, remember that to be a success in the salon profession you must:

- ✄ Plan your work, work your plan, and use your time as if every second counts...because it does
- ✄ Define your plan with a unique selling philosophy
- ✄ Understand the foundation of selling and marketing
- ✄ Retain clients

These aren't easy tasks, but the passionate salon professional does them with determination. Keep in mind as you sharpen your marketing techniques that you are not just selling. You are assisting clients in achieving their personal goals which in turn helps people feel more confident.

As a salon professional you must often wear the two hats of success: The selling hat and the helping hat. It's a juggling at times, but with the information you'll find in the next section on team building, you'll discover that there are many people out there willing to help. And I'm here, right now, to help you, too.

Section 5
Building Your Dream Team

Let's talk teams. The concept of teams goes beyond the networking philosophy of the eighties, and the idea of team building will stretch well into the next decade. As with an athletic team, your personal team is there to help, assist, support and listen. One team member helps another. This is simple and very effective.

Who is included on your team? That's really up to you. Generally, I consider a team to include those individuals who help make your life happen. As the "owner" of your team, the captain, the focal player and a supporter, too, you might have all-star players and possibly a few who rarely show up for practice. And maybe even one or two who gripe throughout the game. Every team is different.

For example, my team includes my husband Bert, our children, families, and friends. It extends to colleagues, support staff and acquaintances. The individual who helps prepare my income taxes is on my team as is the person who cares for our yard.

Because life isn't all black and white, we can't dismiss, fire or trade mediocre players from our teams as they do with the Chargers or the Padres. On our personal team, we realize that people deserve to have their best opportunities presented. Sometimes doing that is up to us. At other times, we must let go of a team member so he or she can get on another's team.

With the information you'll find in this section, you can begin to format a dream team. This team, personally and professionally, will help you achieve the goals of success you've outlined previously or perhaps only aspired to have. Just as you and I are totally different, our teams will not be the same.

When was the last time you gave your team a pep talk or a word of praise? When was the last time you really considered that you're not working alone in this great big world?

In this section, we'll investigate how to honor our team and improve it. We'll start at the bottom with a definition of a team player and work our way up the team ladder. What's the bottom line on team building? I believe it's a working attitude that includes all the basics of the Golden Rule. When you really think of it, isn't the Golden Rule all you really need to follow to achieve success?

Definition of Team Players

1. They have plenty of drive.

2. They accept responsibility cheerfully.

3. They not only welcome responsibility, they seek it.

4. They look, listen, and learn.

5. They find out if they're not sure.

6. They prepare to inspire through their example.

7. They welcome new ideas.

8. They don't expect the credit.

9. They realize the future is their own responsibility.

10. They think things through first.

11. They believe good manners are good business.

12. They set a goal for themselves. They know where they want to go, are willing to study and work in order to get there.

13. They know the world does not owe them a living. They feel they owe the world their best and the world will reward them accordingly.

14. They realize that everything worth having has a price tag. It has to be paid for in personal effort. Nothing is free, not even failure.

15. They earnestly want to succeed.

17. They make others feel important.

18. They always try to help the "boss."

19. They keep their promises.

20. They understand and use the complex simplicity of the Golden Rule.

In case you skimmed over these attributes, they're identical to those held by successful, problem-solving team leaders. How do you fit the image?

> *"Mistakes are easy, mistakes are inevitable, but there is no mistake so great as the mistake of not going on."*
> — William Blake

Building a Solid Foundation

How it works

The concept of team building, the term we'll use rather interchangeably with networking, is simple: It's planning and making contacts. It's sharing information for professional and personal gain and betterment. The key words of that definition are *planning* and *personal*. Team building has to be planned. It doesn't occur when you're least expecting it. A quality team happens only when supportive and friendly relationships, as well as strong, willing business contacts, are built and fortified.

Team building is a 24-hour process that includes *giving as well as getting*. You can't expect to attend one network meeting every six months and get results. Don't be that naive. You must always be on the lookout for people you can include in your network and whose networks you can join. Understand that you may not benefit immediately, but somewhere down the pike you will. It may take years to see the results of your team building...or it may happen overnight with a phone call and a follow up.

We must constantly work to improve our teams. That team will then be there to support us should we suddenly decide to change fields, salons or locations. With team support, you won't have to scramble for a new foundation to assist you; the team's support moves along with you introducing you to new team members.

Set your goals

Look at your business associates and think of their team support. To build a firm foundation for your team, it's essential to decide who you really want to be there for you. More over, you must decide who you want to be there for. You need to know how to contact these people and how they can help you — while you are helping them.

Some people prefer to make phone calls rather than contacting through the mail. Others feel strongly in the opposite direction. I challenge you to work on this hurdle to success. After all, building a foundation for your team to win is all about pushing yourself (you are your product). You must be self-confident.

As you set goals to build a team or a network, consider how your team building "rendezvous" will take place. Will you meet in the salon, at an office, over coffee or lunch, at a friend's home or over the telephone? A less-threatening method to meet new people who will provide a positive addition to your team is by joining networking groups, professional associations and volunteer programs. However, you must attend the meetings and volunteer to be an active part of their committees in order to find new team members. Your goal is to be noticed so that you can notice others who are the movers and shakers of their field.

Samantha, a salon professional in the Denver area, had just moved to that city when we met at a beauty show. Over coffee, she and I talked about this specific topic.

Samantha reported, "Initially, I was flustered about my husband being transferred from Buffalo. I'd worked hard in my hometown to establish a working team and had a great clientele. When I knew the move was forthcoming, I started asking people on my team about the mile-high city.

"Much to my pleasure, I found out that the volunteer branch of the American Cancer Society, that I've worked with for years, has a very active group in the city. Hearing about the move, my attorney called a colleague in Denver and she invited me to join their networking group and attend their chamber's mixers. And then I contacted the product line distributor in Buffalo and asked her to call their rep in Denver. With those team contacts, I instantly had connections. The manufacturer gave me the inside scoop on salons in the area and continuing education. The networking group provided instant clients for my new salon, and through a contact at the volunteer group, I even found after-school care for my kids."

Plan your strategy

If you've been procrastinating, it's past time to make a list of team members who are already in your working network. On a second list, go through your card file and list the people with whom you haven't spoken in six months. Perhaps you want to reconnect with men or women from more than a year ago. List those people, too.

Have you ever read articles or books by some of the "stars" in your specific field or had friends tell you about a wonderful speaker, author or colleague you positively must meet or hear? Many of these people, even the really well-known ones, could be included in your team building program. List them, too. Why? Because they could be an influential contact on your team.

Take action

Set a timetable to achieve your goals. Perhaps you can aim for one cold call or a call to revive an ancient friendship every day, or even once a week. Perhaps you can make two reconnecting lunch or coffee dates a week. Work from your list and make notes of the responses.

Stick with your schedule. Stay on track. Periodically, read over your notes. You're going to be surprised and encouraged by how many contacts you are making. You'll be heartened by how strong your team is becoming.

Many salon professionals find that it helps to set aside a special team-building time. I use Mondays since that's one of the days I'm not in the salon. Another individual might use the early part of Sunday evening to make telephone calls to stay connected to a team. That's a smart move, too, especially if some of the contacts require a long-distance call.

When going to any type of meeting, wisely distribute a certain number of your business cards. Make the second goal to collect cards from those individuals you believe may have a significant impact on your team.

Just do it

Certainly, you may feel awkward at first. But I promise you the more you talk with people about business, the more comfortable it will become. Here's a special tip: Ask new acquaintances questions that require their opinion. People love to talk about themselves and the information they provide during the conversation will help you determine if you want to add them to your team.

I still get nervous when I enter a new networking environment. Now I use this fear or nervousness as a barometer that I'm going in the right direction.

For instance, you might ask when first meeting someone, "I've heard you've been a salon owner for ten years. What meaningful changes do you foresee in the future in our area?" Needless to say, this person will be able to talk about that for a minimum of five minutes. What's the benefit? You have the opportunity to find out a lot about this salon owner in the course of that time, determine if you'd like him or her on your team, plus gain a bit of new insight on your profession.

One caution here: Don't become a slave to your network. Be selfish — it's okay. Work toward making your network and your team support your goals and in turn, work to help support others.

From Cold to Hot: Tips on Getting Your Team Together

At various times in life, we've all felt strange about talking to new people — some of us more than others. Here are some sure-fire tips to get through those first few dreaded minutes and help you build your team and your confidence at the same time.

Prepare

Before arriving at a networking meeting, find out as much as possible about the agenda, as well as the group hosting the event. It's often a good idea to make contact with someone at the group's headquarters beforehand. You might want to ask a question about the speaker or the length of the program when calling the headquarters. What does this do? You'll have established rapport with one individual at the meeting; there will be a friendly face that you can connect with the phone voice.

Psyche up

In any networking opportunity, your attitude is your most important asset. Refocus your preoccupation from your own anxieties to thinking about the others attending the meeting.

Pretend you are about to host a party and concentrate on helping others have a good time. Don't think of the men and women at the event as a frightening, unknown mass of humanity (you'll be overwhelmed). Rather, think of them as individuals to meet on a one-to-one basis.

Research what you'll say

Get your personal introduction down pat. Add a funny remark and smooth out questions you want to ask.

Talk small

Have at least three "small talk" questions in mind to serve as conversation openers. Successful ones include:

"How did you find out about the meeting tonight?"

"What are you hoping to learn from the speaker's talk?"

"Are you a member of the organization? Why did you join?"

Open-ended questions are your best bet when making initial contact. They draw people out and allow you to turn their answers into two-way conversation.

Seek every opportunity to meet people

Don't wait until you actually walk into that meeting or conference to begin building your team. If you arrive at the meeting by car and notice a group heading toward the door, take the opportunity to strike up a conversation.

"Are you going to the women's networking meeting? Did you run into much traffic once you left the highway?" Whether you are at the check-in desk, the elevator, or waiting at the bar, start talking.

Use that name tag

Use the name tag that's always given to your best advantage. Apply it to your right lapel. What difference can it make to put on the right or left side of your suit jacket? Considerable. When you extend your hand to meet someone, that person's eyes move from your hand to your sleeve, to your lapel's name tag and to your face. What you've done is help the person make a connection from your written name to your smiling face.

I recommend that you make your name tag easy to read — be sure to print letters large and make them stand out. You might draw a star next your name, doodle, or underline the letters.

Find kindred spirits

I know it's intimidating at times, but you must make eye contact in order to meet people. Making eye contact is one of the most crucial tools for successful mingling, and thus team building. When you seek out people to talk with, scan the reception area for eye contact and friendly smiles. Likewise, a person who averts his or her eyes and turns away will not easily be approached. Stick with those men and women who, like you, want to build a team.

Additionally, seek out people who are by themselves at a meeting. Instead of heading straight for the laughing group of five gathered around the buffet or bar, find someone who would welcome meeting you, that is, someone who is perhaps looking uncomfortable and standing alone.

What does one say? How about: "Have you tried the appetizers?" "Have you heard the speaker before?" "Are these gatherings usually this crowded?" Take it from there — I'm sure you get the idea.

Seat yourself strategically

If seats are not assigned at the event, use this opportunity to meet more new people. Do not approach a round table where eight people are seated and only one or two seats are left. The group will already be engaged in conversation and may not notice your arrival. However, if you approach a table where only a few people are seated, you'll find them eager and grateful to welcome you.

To break the ice, return to your small talk or openers that you've rehearsed. Don't hesitate to tell the group that this is your first meeting. People are anxious to help newcomers, which leads to new connections for you. This is how I built my business. It's amazing how much fun it is and how easily you gain credibility and friendships.

Keeping Your Team in the Game

You can't just build a team and then walk away, never to maintain it. Teams fall apart that way and your hard work could be lost. Here are a few ways to preserve a strong network.

Be organized

All your contacts — all those team members — won't do you any good unless you organize them. Think about how this information will be most helpful to you and then consider your plan.

File 'em

Many people use a multiple-rolodex system to organize their team. The file on top of your desk, they suggest, is for the current contacts. A second business card file contains the names of people you want to gain access to, but know you won't be speaking with more than once every few months, if that. And a third, optional, file contains "old timers," those people with whom you haven't been in contact for more than a year.

Color code 'em

You can organize the network on color-coded or alphabetized index cards, categorizing your contacts and keeping tracks of the calls you make to each. Give your network a check up at least once a year. Weed out and reorganize your card files, rolodexes and address books.

Keep your list of current and active contacts close at hand. Don't discard old but valid contacts; you can always reconnect and may need this team member to provide some information sometime in the future.

Caring for Your Contacts

Maintaining is fine — it's absolutely necessary when you're building a team — but you need to do more. You need to care for your contacts.

Your contacts can open doors for you if you earn their respect by building mutually satisfying relationships. Remember, nobody likes a user or a loser. If you network while you're employed and doing well, if you're concerned about what you can give to your team members, should you need assistance when you're down or require advice, there will always be a hand stretched out to you.

Foster a giving attitude

Call contacts every few months just to say hello. Call and offer your help. For most people, a no-strings-attached phone call from a colleague will be a pleasant surprise. Your genuine concern and support will be reciprocated when you need to call on the team member.

Remember the little things

Beyond birthday, congratulations and thank you notes, continue to stay in touch with your team members. Send colleagues copies of newspaper or magazine articles that you think will be of benefit. Include a short handwritten note that can be as simple as "FYI," or "Thought you'd find this engaging reading." If the article relates to a mutual interest, especially a professional one, your credibility as a team builder and a career-minded individual will be heightened.

Enhance your connections

Let those on your team know of upcoming events or meetings that might be of interest. Ask that their names be placed on professional newsletters. Call them when there's an activity or event in your area that you can attend together.

Broaden your scope

If you hear of an opportunity that sounds perfect for someone on your team, be sure to tell him or her about it. If you are unable to assist a client but certain a team member could, make a referral.

Your team members will remember your generosity and return it.

Team Etiquette

Possibly the most important "rule" for good team building is to make sure you observe proper etiquette. Every sport, including networking, has customs and dictates. Here are a few essentials to keep in mind when building a winning team.

Respect your contacts' names

Give team members the respect that you'd appreciate when making a referral. Get an okay before you make a referral or use a person's name as a referral to another individual.

Keep an eye on the clock

Be sure to call team members and people you'd like on your team at appropriate times. Make sure the times are convenient for them, not just for you. Don't forget about time differences throughout the United States and body-clock differences, too. I have a night owl colleague. I know I call him past eleven any night, and he'll be wide awake. Another team member wakes well before dawn. I dare not call her after eight in the evening, or I might drag her out of bed.

Follow through on your promises — all of them

If someone asks you for the name of a product or a copy of an article that you've talked about, make a note of the request and forward the information as soon as possible. Fill the request in less than a week. It's often helpful to jot the request on the individual's business card so you'll have all the info you need, plus a reminder. Likewise if you offer anything, make sure you follow through.

Stay visible

Even if you haven't committed yourself to supplying information or referrals to one of your contacts, use written and telephone communication to stay visible. Send your contacts holiday cards and info on updates in your field. Ask them to lunch or coffee "for no reason at all." Clip and send articles of interest or a joke from the morning comic strip.

One salon professional in San Diego keeps what she calls a "smile file," with funny articles and jokes she knows her clients will enjoy. I love opening letters from this woman because I'm always sure to get a chuckle out of them.

Think of creative ways to stay in touch. For example, when you're in a imaginative mood, you might jot down 20 ways to stay connected, make a plan to use these connection tools and work at part of your success program.

Thank everyone

Be sure to recognize everyone who helps you and provides leads, contacts and referrals. At any networking meeting, you're bound to come away with at least three ideas or tips you can use or incorporate into your success program.

Thank those who have offered the tips and suggestions, whether they are helpful or not. A one-minute phone call or a brief handwritten note to let them know they're appreciated means a lot. Contacts appreciate the follow up.

A Final Team Challenge

As you work your team plans and set goals to build your business, be aware that making contacts, networking, or team building, whatever you choose to call it, takes time and commitment. It's a challenge.

Always push yourself. Building a winning team isn't for the faint of heart.

Your job is to approach new people at meetings and social situations. You must start the conversation, even if you've had a rotten day or you're in a bad mood. Take the initiative and it will pay off.

Whether you're a novice or an expert, you'll only get as much out of these team building tips as you put into them.

An Open Letter

This letter, in poem format, has been passed around through networking circles since I've been in business. It's just as pertinent today as it was when someone first handed me a copy.

It has been attributed to an independent direct sales associate, but the author's name has been lost. If you created this letter, my thanks. It has inspired greatness in many and made more than a few of us stop and think.

You never know when someone
May catch a dream from you.
You never know when a little word
Or something you may do
May open up the windows
Of a mind that seeks the light.
The way you live may not matter at all,
But you never know — it might.
And just in case it could be
That another's life, through you,
Might possibly change for the better
With a broad and brighter view,
It seems it might be worth a try
At pointing the way to the right.
Of course, it may not matter at all,
But then again — it might.

Making the Right Connections

We all love giving and getting referrals. That's the true role of team building, but have you given thought to the fact that it's the quality of the referral that counts, not the quantity?

Let's talk about qualified referrals, unqualified referrals, inside referrals and outside referrals. Let's concentrate on making the right connections.

A qualified referral is one which is either from yourself or from a client, a friend, business associate or other individual who you know is going to use your product or service. This person should have been contacted. By contacting her before making the referral, she knows she'll be getting a call. Contact with both parties prior to their introduction results in a qualified referral — it gives each person the opportunity to say, "No thanks" ahead of time. It also gives you a great opportunity to stay connected to your own team members. This also allows your associates to really see that you are working for them.

An unqualified referral is one where you believe that someone could use your service. You have an idea that someone could use your products or services and you follow up on it. The referral only becomes qualified when purchase of the product or service is made. There's nothing more awkward than to contact a referral who has no idea who you are and doesn't seem to care. If someone gives me a referral, I ask a couple of questions. I ask: Would you mind calling ahead to say that I will contact him (or her)? Would you mind calling me when that's completed? This accountability helps to ensure your success with the referral. A couple of minutes of planning can save you a lot of time playing telephone tag.

An inside referral comes from someone in your network or business group who provides a product or service. For example, when I need letters written and reports generated, I contact Linda who runs a local secretarial service. When I wanted a new brochure and business cards, I went to a colleague, Jana, who owns a graphic design studio. We all belong to the same networking group so this is called an inside referral.

The outside referral includes those people who are my personal team members. Betty, a neighbor, recommended that her cousin, Tim, attend one of my goal-setting seminars. Tim went to one, and then he recommended the seminars to associates in the large computer software company he owns. This is an outside referral, and outside referrals are everywhere if you only let others know that you are always looking for clients.

Strive to use the resources around you to generate referrals. It is your job to make quality referrals.

For instance, one salon professional I've known forever always chats about how her sister is the best landscaper in the city. She gabs so much that new clients can't wait to get home to call for a consultation. Sounds like a perfect team member and a great way to get referrals, right? Unfortunately, this woman isn't making quality referrals. In actuality, her sister assists corporations by creating environmental green belts; she doesn't work with homeowners at all. What happens in situations such as this one is that the clients who were interested are disappointed. The next referral from this woman will be ignored. Clients won't believe that she's making quality referrals whether it really is one or not.

Make it a personal goal to generate two outside referrals this week. Do this by listening carefully to clients and others on your team. Ask questions. See how you can support someone on your team. People will support what they help create.

"I have found the enthusiasm for work to be the most priceless ingredient in any recipe for success."
— Samuel Goldwyn

Referrals: Worth Their Weight in Gold

Imagine this: You're not a salon professional. It's your birthday, and you're excited and pleased with the prospect of a fun-filled day. There will be surprises and cake and cards and...well, you get the picture. You know your friends and family are planning something; they've been hinting for weeks — well at least you think they have. Ah, that happy birthday feeling is growing and blossoming inside.

Halfway through the day, you haven't received any birthday phone calls. There were no flowers awaiting your return from lunch and no cards cluttering the front desk. Well, maybe there will be a surprise party after work or when you get home.

But when you arrive home, everything is quiet. You open the mail box and along with the assorted bills and an ad or two is a birthday card. It's from your salon professional. Instantly, a smile shines on your face. Somebody remembers and is thinking of you.

Okay, it's just make believe and it would be sad if no one remembered your special day.

This analogy has a purpose. Do you see our integral role in client and team member's lives and the value of the part we play. Looking at the scenario again, just the thought that we've taken time to remember a birthday or other special day stays with the person for weeks, maybe even years.

Let me make this perfectly clear. Working to make your clients satisfied has nothing to do with manipulating or exploiting your relationship, unless you take it to that extreme. Rather, by being considerate and thoughtful you build a reputation for being considerate and thoughtful. People like to buy services from people with whom they enjoy doing business. Really now, wouldn't you prefer a smile to a frown in any business situation?

Remembering personal events of importance is part of the way we let our clients and team members know they are special and important to us. Because they are.

Sue, a client who has been with me for about eight years, worked with me on a project some years back. And when I was recently going through a box of old photos, I found one of us together the night of an awards ceremony. We looked pretty spectacular at the event.

I sent her the photo and a card saying that I just wanted to remind her of how beautiful she is. The next time I saw Sue, she had tears in her eyes. She thanked me for reminding her. The card came when she really needed it.

This little gesture of love and friendship took two minutes. But that little gesture brought Sue and me even closer. Sometimes we forget things as simple as saying: You are special.

Oneida, a salon professional, heard me speak on this topic at a seminar and she immediately put it into practice. Saint Joseph's Day, a religious holiday, holds special significance for some of her clients, and it was coming up in a few weeks. Oneida instantly got the message. After the seminar, she drove directly to the Hallmark shop, bought some cards and sent them. Oneida phoned me a few weeks later. "One of my client's was crying when she called to say how the card touched her. *Then* two of her friends called to make appointments. I may buy stock in Hallmark if this keeps up."

You needn't be fancy with cards — plain and tasteful stationery works great. Let's look at other opportunities to connect with clients:

✂ A simple welcome card following a first time visit

✂ A thinking-of-you card for someone in distress

✂ A congratulations card for a success

✂ A sympathy card during a time of need

✂ An anniversary, retirement or bon voyage card for a special time

Sending cards through the mail is a great marketing tool that costs less than $1.50. And this form of advertising really leaves the client or team member anxious to connect with you again.

The art of staying connected with team members is worth its weight in gold. Extend your thanks, stay connected and make other people feel great. Do you know what? You'll feel better, too. This technique can make a difference in peoples' lives. It's so simple, yet so valuable.

161

Decide to Network

Use every letter you write
Every conversation you have
Every meeting you attend
To express your fundamental beliefs and dreams.
Affirm to others the vision of the world you want
Network through thought
Network through action
Network through spirit
You are the center of a network
You are the center of the world
You are a free, immensely powerful source
of life and goodness.
Affirm it.
Spread it.
Radiate it.
Think day and night about it
and you will see a miracle happen:
The greatness of your own life.
Networking is the new freedom
the new democracy
A new form of happiness.
— by Dr. Robert Muller

Praising Your Team and Your Clients

Have you ever wondered why some salon professionals are more successful than others? Of course. We all have.

So what is it? What makes the difference? Is it the salon? The locale? The manager or the staff? What do the successful salon professionals do that you possibly don't or don't know how to do?

This happens to be one of the hottest topics of conversation at the seminars I conduct. Why so? I believe it is because the weight of praise and how it relates to success is so often misunderstood.

Praise and recognition are ideas that could signify success or setback in your business. They represent two seemingly simple concepts, but I believe many salon professionals dismiss them as too easy.

In my consulting business working with scores of salon professionals, I find that the number one reason why clients do not return for additional products or services is that the professional doesn't seem to appreciate them. A little praise and personal attention can accomplish wonders. With a touch of appreciation, one can increase the client's morale, create more sales, and bring in quality referrals. Isn't that our goal?

Last year, I took a survey among my clients and asked the reason why they kept coming back. I was very surprised with the answer. I thought maybe it was my talent with colors or haircuts. But do you know what? It was because they could feel the love and appreciation I had for them and for my work. I make clients feel special; I make them feel like they are queen for a day. It's pretty amazing what happens when you give away praise and recognition.

There are three types of recognition that we need to be aware of. The first is *cash.* Yes, we're talking about the folding green stuff. Rewarding clients with cash incentives is not tacky — it works. You needn't pass along crisp $100 bills, but rather offer discounts off the total price for purchasing larger services or products. For example, if a client is considering the services of a color, perm, and a cut, it makes great sense to offer a discount on a deep conditioning or another service you provide.

Do you love discounts? Everyone does and they're a great way to give recognition to clients and team members. I offer my clients a 25 percent discount on their next services when they refer me clients. I reward them for contributing to my business. I give them a $100 gift certificate to a terrific restaurant or department store for providing three qualified referrals during a certain period of time.

Let's say ten of my clients take advantage of this offer. Yes, I've spent $1000 to get new clients. However, to add 30 new clients to my books — clients who will spend an average of $200 to $1500 a year — makes my promotional dollars well spent. More so, I didn't have to pay for any advertising. I used my team to help my business and bring a marvelous return on a small investment.

The second item of recognition is verbal acknowledgment. Nothing is sweeter to hear than, "I really appreciate your sending Dr. Jones to me." Honor and recognize the person who makes the referral.

Eddy was just another a Cincinnati-based salon professional dreaming of opening a contemporary salon. That changed when Eddy got a qualified referral from a client to an venture investment banking firm. Eddy and the firm worked out a great business deal, and that dream is now a dream of a salon.

Eddy recently told me, "Just sending a card, a note, and a discount on services didn't seem a sufficient thank you for the woman who helped me achieve a life-long goal." Rather, Eddy sent the client a bouquet of flowers to her office on the first day of every month for an entire year. He explains, "I wanted her to know that she'd changed my life for the better — I wanted to brighten her day as she had brightened my future." Yes, Eddy spent an excess of $500 with this unique approach to recognition, but think for a moment how much that network contact appreciated the continuing thanks, how loyal the client remained, and how many people this client told about the event and Eddy's success story.

Whether we realize it or not, we're often mentors or parent figures to our clients. Thus, it is not unusual that they may look to us for encouragement that they are doing something right. Just like an Olympic athlete needs praise from a coach, our team and our clients need praise and recognition from us.

I challenge you to make praise and recognition one of your goals. Find something that everyone you come in contact with is doing right and congratulate them. For example, perhaps one of your clients has been chosen Business Person of the Year. Let him or her know how proud you are — he or she was just destined for success with all that tenacity and creativity.

You'll have a pleasant surprise if you begin to praise and recognize your clients and team members. They'll start referring clients to you and those clients will refer more. It's a perfect win-win situation, yet it's up to you to begin the cycle.

Third, acknowledge each occasion that benefits a client or team member. Many salon professionals, business owners and other professionals underestimate this powerful way to recognize others. Acknowledgments might include thank you notes, birthday cards, flowers, a gift for the office, a box of chocolates or a basket of fruit. Imagine how I felt not too long ago when a client, Debbie Thomas, gave me a gift basket filled with cookies, gourmet chocolates and big, gold ornaments in it. What do you want to bet that I'll see if I can make another great referral to this team member? I was recognized and my work was acknowledged (and the chocolates were scrumptious). My goal with clients and team recognition is to make each receive some appreciation from me, every time we meet or on all special occasions. I love creating win-win situations and relationships. You can be sure I'm going to mirror that gift basket with my next special thank you.

Use your own unique way with business to create what works best for you. Try this technique for just a few months, and I can guarantee your business will boom.

The effectiveness of the coach reflects the strength of the team. You are the coach so help your team make you all winners. Therefore, if your clients are not giving you the results you desire, maybe it's time for you to re-evaluate your business techniques and your skills as a team member and team builder. Do you have a plan of action? Do you know what you personally would like your team members or your staff to do? Do you know what each client or team member really wants for his or her own business? What are their career goals? What are your own career goals?

These aren't easy questions. Yet, when you have answers to them, you are on your way to a great future, right along with a great team to cheer you on as you succeed.

Your Praise and Recognition Challenge

Here's your challenge: List 50 ways you can praise and offer recognition to your clients. No one is looking over your shoulder so don't be shy. Include incentives like discounts and verbal praise like compliments.

Imagine for the next week that all of your clients and team members are wearing signs that say: "Make me feel important and special."

You've been doing business with the people on your client and team list for some time — you have a relationship. Your job for the next week, therefore, is to give away at least one compliment to each person you meet. Find something unique and special about each of them.

That old adage says: What goes around, comes around. Watch out — not only will you feel great by giving praise and recognition, but you'll get plenty back, too.

Handling Difficult Clients

Problems come up. It's part of our business. There are client complaints and hard-to-get-along-with people in every business and when we're working with the intimate situation of the salon, it's obvious that we'll be faced with problems every once in a while.

Let's take on some of the more trying events and situations starting with "no shows." In the past, perhaps like you, I may have hounded my no show clients. No shows cost salon professionals money and not showing up for an appointment is discourteous, too. But I've switched my philosophy to one that works better so I'm sharing it with you. Rather than calling to rant and rave to clients, call and be concerned. Surely the client would never leave you in the lurch; therefore, something serious must have happened. Sometimes I apologize that I've had a mix-up and hope I haven't inconvenienced them. I "own" the responsibility for my business and for the no shows. Through showing my concern and apologizing should there have been a mix up, I have a much higher response and so fewer no shows, it's incredible. In the past when I'd charge people or complain, I'd end up alienating clients — losing them. My current client base includes busy professionals who must live on hectic schedules. They rarely ever miss an appointment. For those who do intend to flake on appointments, they're not really needed in my client base.

If you're having a lot of no shows, look to yourself. Ask what you are doing that promotes no shows. Do people see you as a professional? Are you on time or close to time with each appointment? Do your clients not see you as someone who values your own time? For instance, if you say, "Hey, no big deal if you don't show," a client will hear exactly that and most likely, not show up for the appointment.

In Summary

Thank you for reading this book and selecting me to help you regain your passion for our business and for your career. Yes, I'm practicing what I preach, and I'm praising you. It's something we should all do naturally, but giving praise and recognition is a habit. All habits (even those bad ones) take about six weeks to become thoroughly established. Make your new positive way to praise a habit, and you'll have learned one of the true secrets of success.

To review what we've discussed in this section, we've talked about:

- ✄ Building a solid foundation
- ✄ Keeping your team in the game
- ✄ Caring for your contacts
- ✄ Practicing team etiquette
- ✄ Making the right connections
- ✄ And of course the essential of praise

In the next section, we'll put it all together. Yes, there's more work to do; but with your burning passion for success, work is joy. Now, let's capture some of that joy.

Section 6
Passion Plus:
Tips, Recommendations and Affirmations

This is the icing-on-the-cake section of the handbook. I've included tips and recommendations that are simply too important to place anywhere else.

In this section, you'll find some affirmations and visualization suggestions to make your life more fulfilling and your career more successful. I know these are big promises, however, from what you've read so far, you know that these ideas work. The methods included in Passion Plus work too.

More to Think About

1. A typical business hears from only 4 percent of its dissatisfied clients. The other 96 percent just quietly go away and 91 percent will never come back. That represents a serious financial loss for salon professionals who don't know how to treat clients and a tremendous gain to those who do.

2. A survey of "Why Customers Quit" found the following:

   ✂ 3 percent move away

   ✂ 5 percent develop other relationships

   ✂ 9 percent leave for competitive reasons

   ✂ 14 percent are dissatisfied with a product

   ✂ 68 percent quit because of an attitude of indifference toward the client by the person providing service, a manager, or a staff member.

3. A typical dissatisfied client will tell a minimum of seven, quite possibly over ten people, about the problem. One in five will tell twenty. It takes twelve positive service incidents to make up for one negative incident.

4. Seven out of ten complaining clients will do business with you again if you resolve the complaint in their favor. If you resolve it on the spot, 95 percent will do business with you again. On average, a satisfied complainer will tell five people about the problem and how it was satisfactorily resolved.

5. The average business spends six times more to attract new clients than it does to keep old ones. Yet client

loyalty is in most cases worth ten times the price of a single purchase.

6. Businesses having low service quality average only a 1 percent return on sales and lose a market share at the rate of 2 percent per year. Businesses with high quality service average a 12 percent return on sales and service and gain market share at the rate of 6 percent per year and charge significantly higher prices.

Conclusions:

✂ It takes work to keep clients, but more work and money to get new ones.

✂ The only place success comes before work is in the dictionary.

Visualizing Success

Would you like to be the best salon professional possible? Using the power of positive suggestion, or visualization, can help you succeed like never before.

Athletes, actors, and lots of other people use visualization to succeed. For example, the actor may use it to mentally give his or her performance. A singer may silently serenade. A salon professional may visualize how it feels to meet a banker for a small business loan, to work with team members for better attitudes in the shop, or other day-to-day activities. I use this technique in the speaking arena as well.

I always knew or visualized I would speak in front of large audiences. Last year, I spoke in front of a staff managers conference in Los Angeles. There were over five hundred people in the audience. I visualized the audience loving the information and having fun. Well, that's exactly what happened during the conference. I had managers standing on their chairs, swirling hand towels over their heads as they chanted, "I am 100 percent committed to my success." We were also dancing in the aisles. After the conference, I realized I had the vision so clear and I had created the space for people to be outrageous and have fun.

Here's all you need to do...the operative word, however, is *do* because you must make up the visualization in your mind and then replay it a number of times. You are allowed to change the situation, but it always must be positive and affirmative.

Sitting in a comfortable chair or lying on the bed, close your eyes and breathe deeply for a moment or two. Some people find that concentrating on the basic act of inhaling and exhaling, and not thinking of other things, helps prepare their mind. Others listen to music; some read religious or inspirational material. The basic goal in this phase is to relax.

Those who successfully practice visualization often concoct an elaborate relaxation scene. They suggest that visualizing is best when they totally get their minds off daily stress so they concentrate on being in a forest near a running stream. They recommend pretending that one is sitting at the beach or seeing the land from a hot-air balloon. They really concentrate on their "quiet spot," and thus, can get back into it quickly when they need to reduce the tension in their lives as well as use it for visualization.

After a few minutes of relaxation, think in your mind about your situation and walk through it. See yourself as articulate, strong, vital and successful. See a positive outcome of your situation. Make sure you're smiling and feeling powerful. After you've played the scene in your head, do it again. You'll want to repeat the visualization a number of times.

Many experts on the power of positive suggestion believe that our unconscious minds can be "tricked" into believing that because we've visualized a situation, we've physically done it before. That's why performers and athletes find visualization so useful. The second time we do something, it's always easier.

When I have a tough situation, such as managing a temperamental staff member, I always use visualization. I "see" the positive resolution and I see everyone satisfied with the conclusion. Yes, I still have to go through the nasty time, but having that dress rehearsal always makes me feel more confident.

Now it's your turn. I invite you to visualize the positive result of a difficult or complex situation. I challenge you to do it now.

Affirmations

To affirm means to vow, attest, confirm, and establish. Those who are successful in the salon industry often use personal affirmations when they are changing or modifying their behavior. I believe in affirmations; we can't get enough positive feedback, and when we hear ourselves say things that are positive, we truly do believe them.

Here are some of the positive affirmations I use. Select five, print them on a sheet of paper and make them part of your day.

- ✄ The responsibility for me is with me. I am not responsible for what happens out there, what others think or what others do. I am responsible only for how I *choose* to respond.

- ✄ Obstacles are what I see if I take my eyes off the goal.

- ✄ Some succeed because they are destined to. Most succeed because they are determined to. I fit into this second group.

- ✄ It's funny about life. Refusing to accept anything but the best, often results in just that. I refuse to accept anything but the best.

- ✄ The trouble with many is that they stop trying in trying times. I refuse to stop trying.

176

Promises for Well-Being

I promise:

1. To understand that the beliefs I have about myself and others may make me feel sad, guilty or inadequate. These are beliefs and may or may not be based on fact.

2. To remember that I am an adult. Adults have power.

3. To understand that I am not a child. I am not helpless.

4. To be aware that I have choices, I have freedom and I have the ability to change.

5. To be conscious that my self-esteem is important. I have the opportunity every day to build my self-esteem for my own good.

6. To be thoughtful as I surround myself with loving, nourishing and supportive people.

7. To take responsibility for my actions, even if they happen to be thoughtless, cruel, victimizing, or hurtful.

8. To stop trying to manipulate others with my behavior, attitudes or actions.

9. To confront people in my life who have caused injury and to address the issues.

10. To deal with those who have hurt me and work toward a more honest relationship.

11. To be aware that I may remove hurtful people from my life, whomever they may be. Adults have power to do so.

12. To recognize that there may be times in my life when I'm depressed, overwhelmed, lonely and sad. The feelings that emotions bring are natural and part of living; they are not scary and should be faced.

13. To seek professional help if these periods continue for longer than necessary.

14. To know that reaching out for help takes courage and honesty and that I am a courageous and honest individual.

In Summary

Just because we've finished with the topics shared within these pages, doesn't mean an end to our relationship. I want to believe that we're team members — and in fact, it's true because we both want the same things on our journey. We want success and passion.

I hope you'll stay in touch. You can use the address below to contact me and give feedback, to share your successes, and just to say hello. Remember when I told you I love getting mail. It's true, so don't hesitate to write.

My final words of encouragement are offered with love, hope and respect. My wish, my prayer, is that you will recapture and define your passion. Through the process, I hope you will also discover happiness.

Address: Susie Fields & Associates
2713 Loker Avenue West
Carlsbad, California 92008

Recommended Reading

Here are a few of the books and tapes that have had special significance for me and other salon professionals.

Ailes, Roger. *You Are the Message: Getting What You Want by Being Who You Are.* New York: Doubleday, 1988.

Bell, Chip R. *Customers as Partners: Building Relationships That Last.* San Francisco: Berrett-Koehler Publishers, 1994.

Boe, Anne. *Is Your Net Working?* New York: John Wiley & Sons, 1989.

Brown, Charlene. *The Consumer's Credit Book: How to Repair or Get Credit.* Irvine, California: United Resources Books, 1991.

Burley-Allen, Madelyn. *Listening: The Forgotten Skill.* New York: John Wiley & Sons, 1982.

Clason, George. *Richest Man in Babylon.* New York, Plume, 1989.

Drummond, Mary-Ellen. *Fearless and Flawless Public Speaking.* San Diego: Pfeiffer & Co., 1993.

Dyer, Wayne. *You'll See It When You Believe It.* New York, William Morrow, 1989.

Gitomer, Jeffrey. *The Sales Bible.* New York: William Morrow, 1994.

Griffith, Joe. *Speaker's Library of Business Stories, Anecdotes and Humor.* Englewood Cliffs, New Jersey: Prentice Hall, 1990.

Gschwandtner, Gerhard. *Non Verbal Selling Power.* New York: Prentice Hall, 1985.

Hardy, C. Colburn. *Retire Prosperously.* Englewood Cliffs, New Jersey: Prentice-Hall, 1990.

Lassen, Ali. *Power Plays: Getting the Edge on Your Competition Through Focused Networking.* Carlsbad, California: Ali Lassen's Success Systems, 1992.

Lorier, Terri. *The Source Book: Essential Resources for Independent Entrepreneurs.*

Pesce, Vince. *A Complete Manual of Professional Selling: The Modular Approach to Sales Success.* Englewood Cliffs, New Jersey: Prentice Hall, 1989.

Savage, Terry. *Terry Savage Talks Money: The Common-Sense Guide to Money Matters.* Chicago: Longman Financial, 1990.

Schneider, Bejamin and David E. Bowen. *Winning the Service Game.* Boston: Harvard Business School Press, 1995.

Wall, Ginita. *Our Money, Our Selves.* Yonkers, New York: Consumer's Union, 1992.

Waitley, Dennis. *Seeds of Greatness.* Old Greenwich, Conn.: Listen USA!, 1983.

Order Form

Fax orders:	(760) 929-2611 (24 hours a day)
Telephone orders:	(760) 929-2600
Postal orders:	Salon Training International, Inc.
	2713 Loker Avenue West
	Carlsbad, California 92008
Website orders:	www.salontraining.com

Please send me:

___ copies of ***Passion: The Salon Professional's Handbook for Building a Successful Business***. For each copy requested, I have enclosed $19.95

Company Name _____

Address _____

City/State/Zip _____

Sales Tax:
Please add $7^{1}/_{2}\%$ for books shipped to California addresses

Shipping:
Book rate: $3.00 for the first book and $1.00 for each additional book. (Surface shipping may take 3-4 weeks.)

Air mail: $4.00 for the first book and $1.00 for each additional book.

Payment:
___ Check   ___Visa   ___ MasterCard   ___Discover

Card Number _____

Name on card_____   Exp. date___ / ___

Call and Order Now!

Order Form

Fax orders: (760) 929-2611 (24 hours a day)

Telephone orders: (760) 929-2600

Postal orders: Salon Training International, Inc.
2713 Loker Avenue West
Carlsbad, California 92008

Website orders: www.salontraining.com

Please send me:

____ copies of *Passion: The Salon Professional's Handbook for Building a Successful Business*. For each copy requested, I have enclosed $19.95

Company Name _____

Address _____

City/State/Zip _____

Sales Tax:
Please add $7^1/_2\%$ for books shipped to California addresses

Shipping:
Book rate: $3.00 for the first book and $1.00 for each additional book. (Surface shipping may take 3-4 weeks.)

Air mail: $4.00 for the first book and $1.00 for each additional book.

Payment:
____ Check ____ Visa ____ MasterCard ____ Discover

Card Number _____

Name on card _____ Exp. date ___ / ___

Call and Order Now!